Optometry *in* America

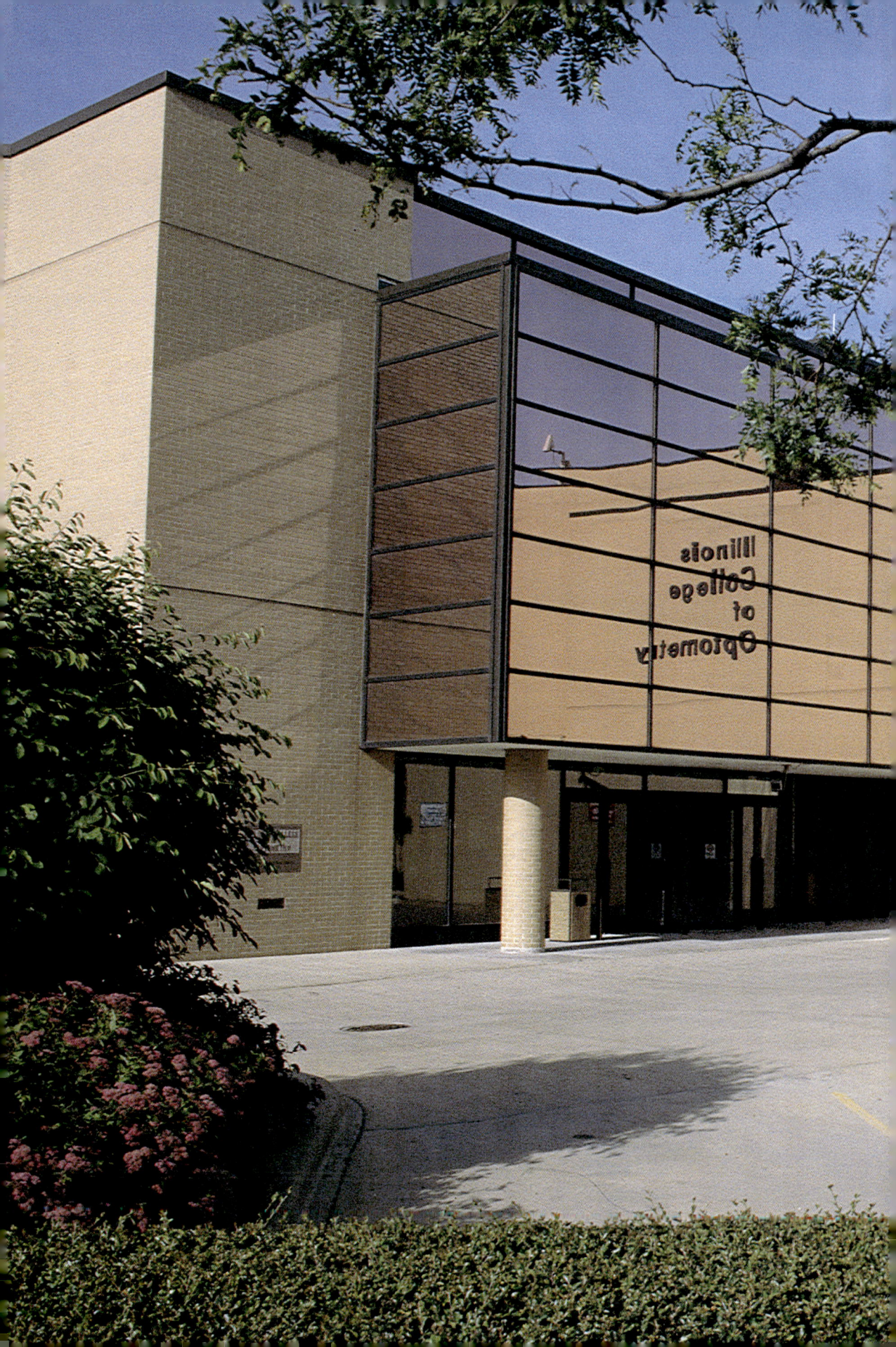

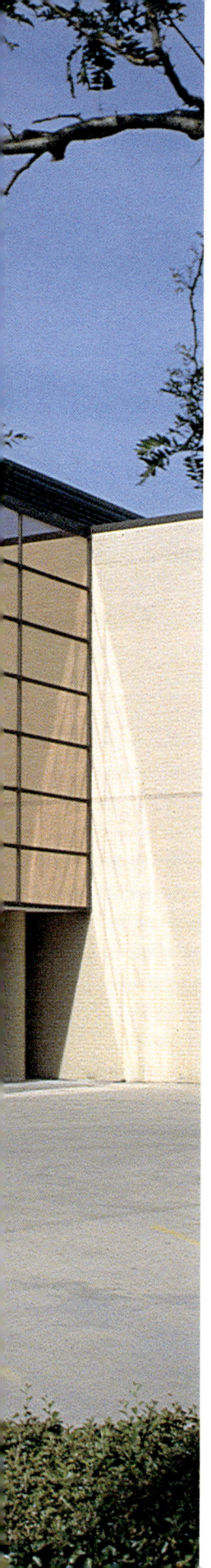
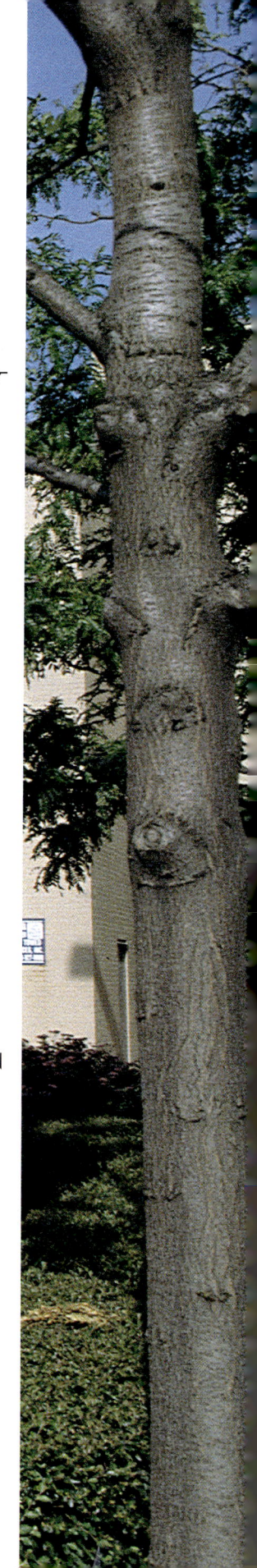

Optometry
in
America

A HISTORY OF THE
ILLINOIS COLLEGE OF OPTOMETRY
1872-1997

ANISTATIA R MILLER & JARED M. BROWN

FOREWORD BY DR. BOYD B. BANWELL

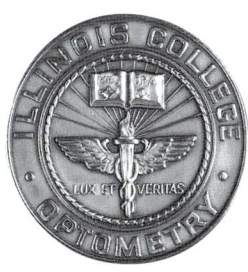

ILLINOIS COLLEGE OF OPTOMETRY
CHICAGO, ILLINOIS

First published in 1996 by
Illinois College of Optometry
3241 South Michigan Avenue, Chicago IL 60616 USA.

Copyright © 1996 by Anistatia R Miller and Jared M. Brown.

All rights reserved.
No part of this book may be reproduced, stored in or introduced into a retrieval system, or transmitted in any form or by any means (including electronic, mechanical, photocopy) whatsoever without written permission from the above publisher of this book, except by reviewers who may quote brief passages to be printed in a magazine or newspaper.

ISBN #: 0-9652759-1-4
Lirbary of Congress Catalog Card Number: 96-77258

Printed in Tokyo, Japan by
Dai Nippon Printing Co., Inc.

CONTENTS

Foreword by Dr. Boyd B. Banwell — vi
Preface & Acknowledgments — viii

CHAPTER ONE
THE QUEST FOR BETTER VISION
The Origins of the Optometric Profession — 1

CHAPTER TWO
THE LARGEST AND BEST EQUIPPED IN THE WORLD
Northern Illinois College of Ophthalmology & Otology — 17

CHAPTER THREE
BRING ON YOUR STATE BOARDS!
Northern Illinois College of Optometry — 41

CHAPTER FOUR
EYES RIGHT
Chicago College of Optometry — 65

CHAPTER FIVE
A NEWER WORLD TO SEE
The Birth of the Illinois College of Optometry — 81

CHAPTER SIX
THE FLAGSHIP
Illinois College of Optometry's Present and its Future — 105

APPENDICES
Chronology — 129
Board of Trustees — 134
Alumni Assocation Members — 135
AOA Presidents — 136
Honorary Degrees and Alumni Awards — 137

Notes — 139
Index — 147
Colophon — 150

FOREWORD

SINCE THE LATE 1800s, when the profession emerged from jewelry stores across the United States of America, optometry has risen from its horse and buggy roots to a previously inconceivable level of sophistication and technology.

In the past century there have been incessantly increasing demands on vision with its relationship to all human functions, which in turn affects how individuals adapt to their environment, occupations, avocations and educational experiences. Optometry is the only profession dedicated to providing necessary care in all of these areas. As such, the field has evolved — meeting these challenges by providing the requisite academic and clinical training in health and vision care.

For me, optometry has provided the opportunity to practice health care in the best interests of the patient — in private practice and co-managed programs with professionals from other health care specialties. Caring for the gift of sight, God's second most precious gift after life itself, has been a truly gratifying experience.

As a practitioner, it has been my responsibility to care for the very young patient with strabismus; the elementary school child with poor grades; and the athlete whose imperfect vision and lack of proper eye/hand coordination were blocks to optimal performance. Some of my most rewarding experiences have been caring for senior citizens whose visual difficulties prevented them from renewing their driver's licenses. It's said that the best form of help is giving someone the means to help themselves, and that's exactly what optometrists do. They enable people to be self-sufficient.

Even with the omniscence of retrospection, I wouldn't exchange my thirty years in independent private practice for any other occupation. I derived great satisfaction not only from helping those with visual problems, but also from participating in optometric legislative activities on the local, state, and national levels. I will always remember the opportunity I had to work with state legislators and members of the Michigan Optometric Association in establishing the Ferris State College of Optometry. That was one of the most exciting experiences of my life. But the pinnacle of my career was becoming President of the very first optometry school ever established in the United States: Illinois College of Optometry.

FOREWORD

As President, I've been able to share three decades of experience with young people entering the profession, and to build a cohesive team at the College — uniting a dedicated faculty, student body, support staff, department directors, administration, and Board of Trustees. This team has set an example for optometric education and clinical care, and for all of higher education. No one could ask for better than that.

It was equally gratifying to work with Governor Jim Edgar of Illinois, Senate President "Pate" Philip, Speaker of the House Lee Daniels, and Representative Frank Watson, the principal sponsor, in the passage of Senate Bill 185 which established new guidelines and responsibilities for the optometric profession in Illinois and throughout the nation.

Since 1872, ICO and its predecessor institutions have led the development of optometry in America. The progression from yesterday's refracting optician to today's optometrist — who provides full-scope patient care through the continued change in optometric didactic and clinical education — has been unprecedented. ICO continues to maintain a leadership position in the development of the profession. As stated in the 1995 Accreditation Report by the Council on Optometric Education of the American Optometric Association, "The [Accreditation Review] team was…impressed by the degree to which the college has been sensitive and responsive to the threats and opportunities presented by the current economic environments in higher education and health care economics."

Optometry is a comparatively young profession. As a result of its rapid augmentation, changes are often misunderstood or pass unseen by other health care providers and patients. Therefore it is important to develop an educational process to better inform the public and other health care professionals as to the role of optometrists in health care. This book, written in plain language by laymen for professionals and non-professionals alike is a step in that direction.

To see its growth and future development, one must look at the history of the profession and ICO's role. It is paramount that our society understands why it is in the public's best interest that optometry continues its aggressive and significant development throughout the next century.

Dr. Boyd B. Banwell
President, Illinois College of Optometry, 1982-1996

PREFACE & ACKNOWLEDGMENTS

BEHIND EVERY BOOK, there is another: the story of its creation, and the many people without whose efforts and devotion, there could never be a final product. To this collection of remarkable people whose knowledge and insights aided in the creation of both the manuscript and this final bound book, we are grateful. First, there was Dr. James B. Hasler who donated his time and talents over the years, gathering many of the historic information resources used in the writing of this volume. Dr. Hasler also conducted critical and timely interviews with the late Judge Morton Abram, Dr. Frederick R. Kushner, Dr. James H. Grout, Dr. Richard Needles, Dr. C.K. Hill, Dr. Walter Yasko, Dr. Alfred Rosenbloom, Jr., and Dr. Irwin Borish.

We are most thankful to the ladies and gentlemen who are the past, present and future of ICO. Dr. Boyd B. Banwell gave us the opportunity to work on this project. His faith, consideration, and support during the research and writing for the school's history made this all possible. In addition, Dr. Banwell tirelessly fielded our questions and gave of his valuable time for interviews. Gerald Dujsik gave us free run of school's libary resources. Al Pouch allowed us to dig through his extensive photographic archives and other illustrative materials. Dr. Mary Flynn gave us a crash-course in clinical procedure at the Illinois Eye Institute. Dr. Walter Yasko aided with the identification of key people and events found in the photographic archives. Barbara B. Renard did an outstanding job as our project liaison throughout the course of development and production. Besides keeping everyone and everything on schedule, she patiently handled the gruelling task of fielding our constant questions. Her guidance and patience were invaluable.

During the finalization of this historical record, a number of readers gave of their time to evaluate its content. We wish to thank Dr. Frederick Kushner, Dr. C.K. Hill, Dr. Walter Yasko and Rita Syzmanski for reading and evaluating the manuscript's content from from their invaluable perspective as long time associates of the school.

Nancy Brown and Brian Morgan read the manuscript in great detail, contributing critical commentary from the layman's point of view. For their insights, we are truly grateful. And without the constant and unfailing support of our agent Lew Grimes, no project would ever find its beginning or its conclusion.

During the design and production of this project, a number of people helped us realize the important visual and physical aspects including Junichi Iwama, Becky Bunting, and the entire production staff of Dai Nippon Printing Co., Inc., whose mastery of their art brought these pages to life; and Anna Pappalardo, Allison Cronin, and Kim Farmer of the Museum of Anthropology at the University of British Columbia.

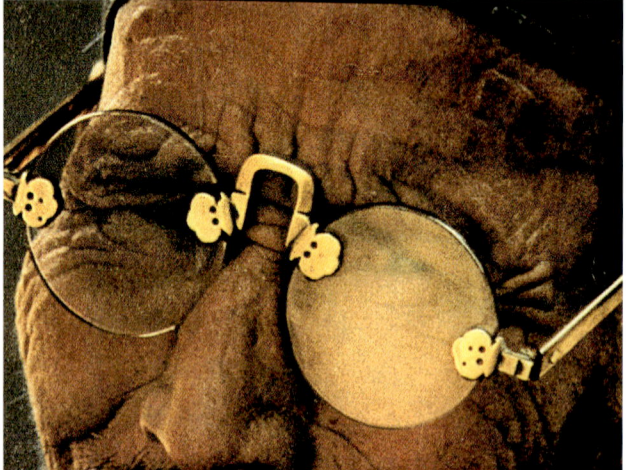

CHAPTER 1

The QUEST *for* BETTER VISION

THE ORIGINS OF OPTOMETRY

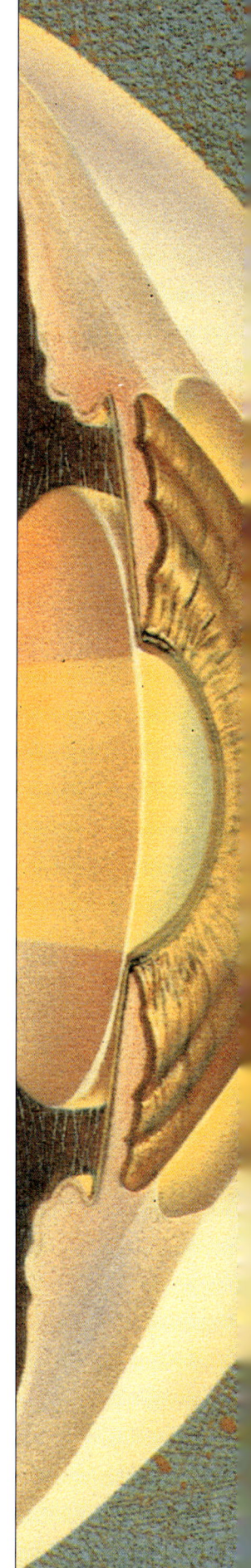

Mankind has sought solutions to vision problems for centuries, using everything from diets and herbs to potions and incantations. Italian explorer Marco Polo reported the use of rock-crystal lenses to magnify print in thirteenth-century China.

OPTOMETRY is America's third largest independent health-care profession. How important is optometry? In our aging society, many people accept that if they don't already wear glasses, they'll probably need them eventually. In much the same way, people just a few centuries ago accepted that if they lived long enough they were likely to lose their eyesight.

As providers of an essential primary health care service, optometrists have been instrumental throughout this century in improving not only human vision but the general quality of life. People no longer have to live with debilitating developmental and educational deficits in childhood, or limited lifestyles as adults and senior citizens because of vision dysfunctions caused by physiological problems, disease, or injury. Many conditions are now easily corrected without surgery or other invasive treatments.

North Americas' oldest and largest optometric college, Illinois College of Optometry — the leader in optometric education — has trained and educated optometrists, since 1872, to become independent primary health care providers who not only examine, diagnose, treat and manage eye diseases and vision disorders, but are capable of diagnosing related systemic conditions in which vision problems are often an early symptom. During its 125-year history, optometry has grown more than in all the previous centuries since the source of human vision was first discovered.

But to gain an understanding of the profession and its educational institutions, it is necessary to begin with roots that extend back thousands of years. Many of the factors that shaped modern optometry — comprehension of the human eye and the source of vision, developments in glass-making, the birth of the science of optics, and conflicts with the medical community — began long before the twentieth century.

PUTTING WORDS TO PAPER

THE INVENTION of the Gutenberg Printing Press, in 1445, could be considered the event that spurred the nineteenth-century development of modern optometry. Improvements in paper manufacturing coupled with Gutenberg's invention made it possible to deliver the written word to a larger audience by packing thousands of words onto a single sheet of paper and reproducing them faster than one page per hour — the approximate amount of time it took a scribe to reproduce a single page of text. Civilization progressed as written communication became portable.[1]

Prior to that, medieval handwritten and illuminated manuscripts were the cutting edge of publishing technology. These beautiful books were extremely expensive and time-consuming to produce, so they were virtually inaccessible to anyone other than the church and royalty.

The first printing presses introduced more books to an affluent lay audience seeking to expand their personal

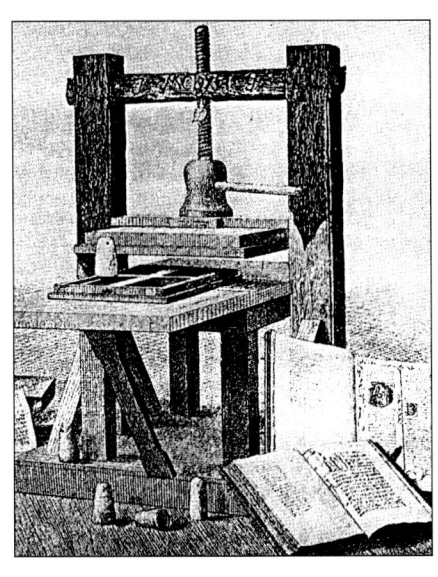

The Gutenberg Printing Press revolutionized the manufacture of books. These new Renaissance status symbols helped trigger a search for improved vision among the well-read elite classes.

ocularii: the Latin name given to eye specialists.

knowledge of numerous subjects including science and medicine. As fifteenth-century physicians and scientists investigated the human body and published their discoveries, they began to realize the increased importance of human vision. Blurred, nearsighted, and farsighted vision existed prior to the Renaissance, but it wasn't until printed books became status symbols among the upper and newly-created merchant classes that vision correction was actively sought.

Before 1300 A.D., people generally accepted their vision problems: they had no alternative. Certain eye diseases were treated by physicians or healers, but most vision defects were not understood and were "corrected" by bloodletting, applying potions and drugs, performing radical skull surgery, or — as in some cases treated by the Roman *ocularii* — by prescribing a physical exercise and dietary program. In other cultures, patients afflicted with vision problems were treated by priests who acted as both spiritual and physical healers. Prayers to the gods were said over the patient to remove their curse or invading evil spirit. Needless to say, the priests' success rates were dismal and people generally chose to live with their impaired vision rather than subject themselves to treatment.[2]

The magnifying properties of glass were discovered more than 4500 years ago by ancient Phoenicians, Egyptians, Greeks, and Chinese, but there is little record of its use in optical enhancement until *The Book of Optics* was written by Arabian scientist Ibn al-Haitham (Alhazen) in 1038 A.D. Alhazen's treatises on light and optics

THE QUEST FOR BETTER VISION

The Chaldean-designed Nineveh lens is made of highly-polished glass. Convex on one side, concave on the other, no one is certain if it was used to ignite fires or to magnify objects.

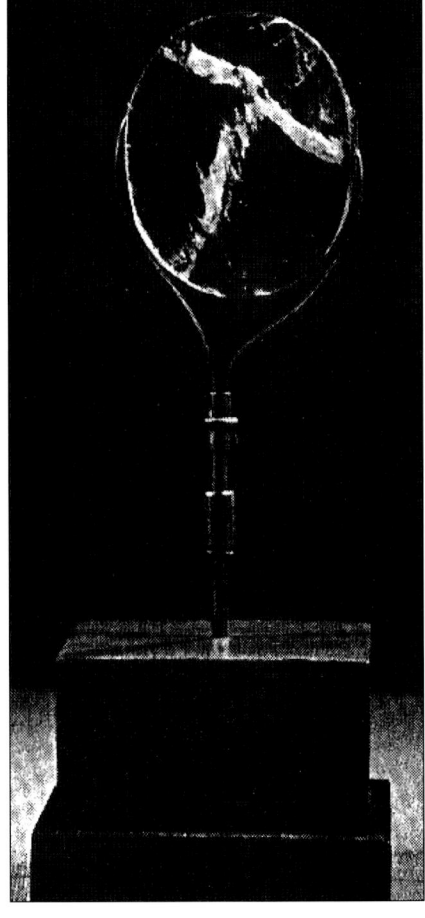

introduced the world to some relevant concepts on the source of human vision, and the ability of convex glass to correct vision flaws. His theories were based on observations made by Euclid and Aristotle in ancient Greece.[3]

Virtually every ancient scientist (including Galen and Ptolemy) and subsequent medieval theoreticians hypothesized on or experimented with refraction and questioned the source of human vision. In the accounts of his thirteenth-century Asian travels, explorer Marco Polo wrote of observing the Chinese reading fine print with rock-crystal magnifying glasses and wearing smoky-quartz-lensed spectacles to shield their eyes from bright sunlight. There were also references to the wearing of spectacles in Ming dynasty (c. 1368-1640 A.D.) texts. The Chinese had even developed a few eccentric social taboos about when and where spectacles could be worn: for example, they could not be worn in front of one's superiors or friends. And the emperor could never be seen wearing spectacles no matter how bad his vision was: it implied that the "Son of Heaven" was imperfect. In western civilization, however, the correlation between the refractive qualities of lenses and human vision had not yet been made.[4]

No one is really too sure who the first western inventor of spectacles was, but by the 1200s European inventors Roger Bacon (who described convex-lensed spectacles in his *Opus Major* (1268)), Salvino d'Armati, and Brother Alessandro della Spina were all credited with the invention of convex-lens spectacles for the correction of presbyopia. But there's no doubt it was this breakthrough that took corrective lenses from theory to actuality.[5]

The invention of concave lenses for correction of myopia probably occurred during the late fifteenth century. Evidence to support this claim can be seen in the Italian artist Raphael's portrait of Pope Leo X (1517): the pontiff wore spectacles for his sitting and the reflections off the glass imply a concave shape. Spectacles with concave lenses were also mentioned by Nicholas Causanus (1401-1464) in his book *De Berillo*.[6]

Early Chinese spectacle frames came in many shapes, from these tie-ons to hinged wrap-around versions.

convex lens: a lens with a convexly curved surface which is used to correct farsightedness.

presbyopia: the decreasing ability to focus on nearby objects due to natural aging.

myopia: a condition where nearby objects can be clearly seen, but there is difficulty in focussing on distant objects (nearsightedness).

concave lens: a lens with a concavely curved surface which is used to correct nearsightedness.

monocle: a single lens — with or without a frame — which is worn by holding it between the brow and cheek.

pince-nez: spectacles without sides which are held on the nose by tension from springs attached to the nose pads.

lorgnette: spectacles that are held in front of the eyes by a handle into which the lenses may fold when not in use.

During the Renaissance, many members of the upper classes and royalty sported monocles, pince-nez, and lorgnettes. These spectacle styles had become exceptionally popular fashion accessories in both France and England. Some people even ordered spectacles with frames made of elaborately-worked leather, shell, horn, or bone — but without lenses.[7]

LOYALTY TO THE CRAFT

UNTIL THE LATE thirteenth century, the majority of technological and scientific discoveries originated from and were spread throughout the known world by travelling monks and clergy. Both the science of optics and the spectaclemaker's art were among the skills shared by this mobile religious community. For this reason alone, it is assumed that many early spectaclemakers were monks.[8]

During the Middle Ages, masons (skilled stoneworkers) also travelled throughout Europe building cathedrals, abbeys, castles, colleges, and other monumental structures. Often working far from any town, workers stayed in masons' lodges near the construction site; and had secret signs or words to prove their *bona fides* to prospective employers. The masons pledged their loyalty to the established customs and usages of their craft. They were bound together by common skills: brothers in a world that didn't welcome strangers. The masons shared their trade secrets among themselves, and only selectively imparted their knowledge to newcomers.[9]

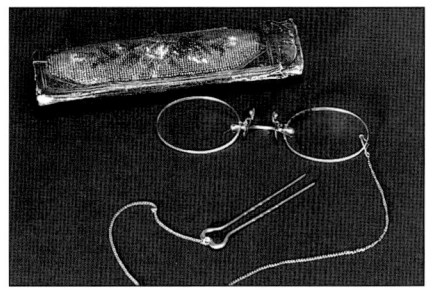

Eyewear was a popular Renaissance fashion accessories. People with perfect vision would order frames with clear lenses.

Many other crafts guarded their trade secrets in a similar fashion. Craft guilds that regulated and standardized the production of goods and performance of services formed all over Europe after the tenth century. The guilds performed the same functions as the masonic brotherhoods: providing illness and burial insurance benefits, maintaining an altar to their particular patron saint, and establishing guidelines of ethical conduct for their constituency. (The major dissimilarity between the masonic societies and the guilds was that unlike the masons, guildsmen generally lived and worked in one town or village throughout their lives.)[10]

Craft guilds eventually became the main spectacle producers. Formed in 1483, The Optical Guild of Regensburg, Bavaria, was one of many German guilds dedicated to spectaclemaking. The guild published their guidelines, detailing group-approved styles and standards of acceptable spectacle design and production. This style guide also contained descriptions of the educational requirements needed to attain levels of craft expertise: from apprentice and journeyman to master craftsman.[11]

For over 200 years, locally controlled and managed guilds regulated the quality of all manufactured goods. Almost every tangible item — from books and wooden barrels to fabric and spectacles — was created by guildsmen. As guild members, spectaclemakers were required to work through a 7-year indentured apprenticeship, a 2-year journeyman or fellowship program, and a master examination in which the applicant created a personal masterpiece: a pair of perfectly crafted spectacles. If the applicant passed the scrutiny of his examiners, he was then granted full membership with the right to select and train his own apprentices.[12]

Other crafts that eventually became health care professions also developed within the guild system's structure. Surgeons who engaged in operative procedures and prescribed treat-

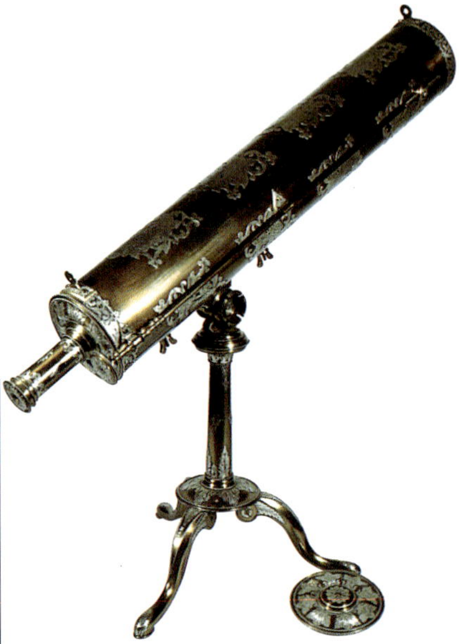

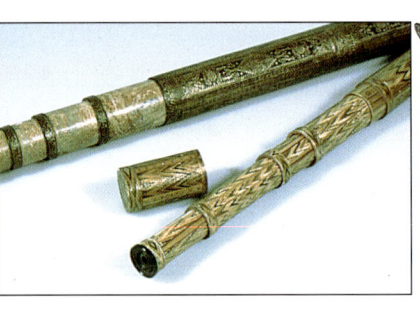

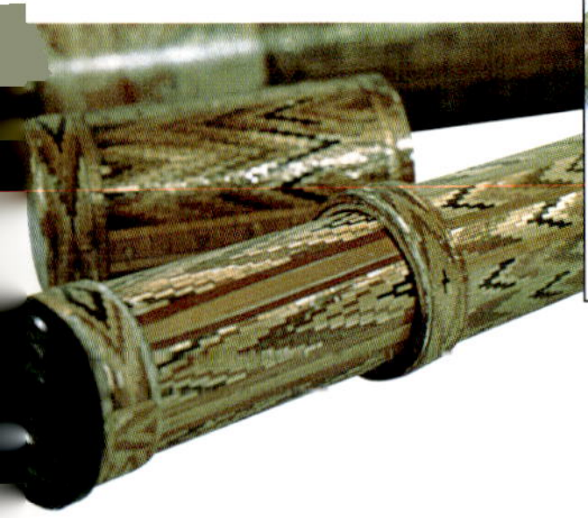

Ornately designed spyglasses and telescopes were also produced by spectaclemakers' guilds.

ments were members of the various barber guilds. Druggists who examined patients, prescribed courses of treatment, and compounded medications were apothecary guild members. The physician-craftsmen who observed and speculated on human disease and prescribed treatment were members of the medical "estates" (another form of guild). Three years of apprenticeship and 2 lecture terms followed by examinations and preparation of a thesis, were required before the title of M.D. and full medical estate membership was awarded.[13]

Over the centuries, the political and economic strength of the European guilds grew. By the 1600s, there were 69 guilds in London alone, including The Master and Court of the Worshipful Company of Spectaclemakers (whose bespectacled patron saint was St. Jerome). Generally speaking, the guilds provided some measure of standardization and professionalism. But unfortunately, the system also fostered a climate of enforced protectionism and isolationism. For example, the Nuremberg High Council prohibited journeymen from leaving their town to work in other places, whereby they could have expanded their knowledge of their given craft.[14] Spectacles made by outside craftsmen were considered contraband by local governments. Imported goods (even those from a neighboring town) were confiscated and heavy fines were levied on offending members for "malpractice." A guildsman who did not strictly adhere to local procedures also had his work confiscated by the authorities; lost the right to work at his craft; and lost his guild membership. In a time when a man apprenticed in his father's trade or was sold into indentured servitude to another master craftsman, this penalty for unconventional behavior meant exile and lifelong dishonor.[15]

Technical advancements fell under similar strictures. New materials or processes that lent a manufacturing advantage to one guildsman over his peers were likely to meet with guild opposition. Plano-convex lens construction, for example, was bitterly opposed by many guilds when it was first introduced because members resisted learning a new technique that radically differed from conventional biconvex lens construction. According the guild's by-laws, it meant educating and recertifying the entire guild.[16]

plano-convex lens: a lens with one plane and one convexly curved surface.

bi-convex lens: a lens with 2 convexly-curved surfaces.

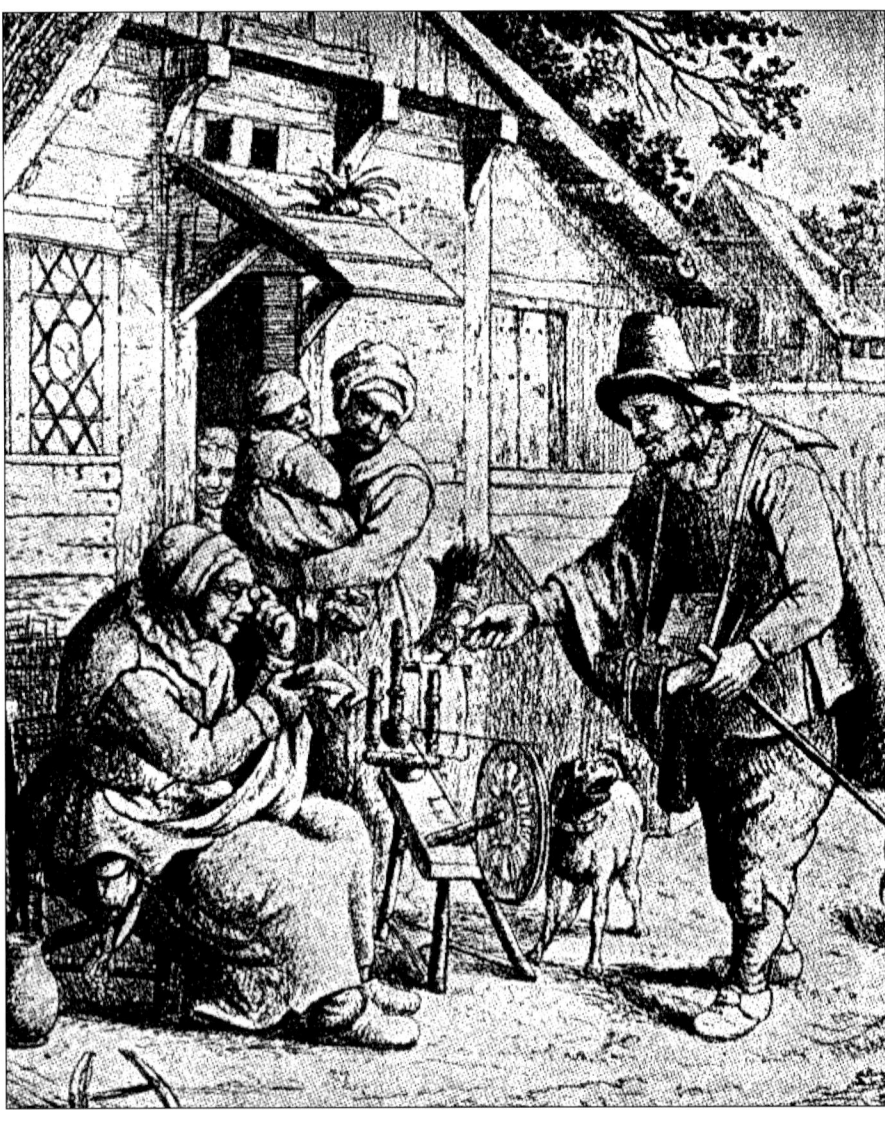

European lens peddlers sold optical goods from town to town as depicted in this drawing by Flemish artist Adrian Van Ostade.

Even though guildsmen were the only people allowed to manufacture lenses, anyone was permitted to fit and sell locally-produced spectacles, and in some cases, even imported ones. At first, the spectaclemakers themselves did not attempt to help purchasers select appropriate spectacles; a customer tried on various lens strengths until he found one that suited him. But by the 1650s, some guildsmen operated their own retail establishments, selling spectacles along with other new optically-based inventions like telescopes and microscopes. Applying their optical expertise, these spectaclemakers were able to fit customers with appropriate lenses more capably than competing vendors — including the door-to-door lens peddlers who hawked their wares to both urban and rural clientele.[17]

MAN HAS TWO EYES — HE NEEDS NOT FOUR

PHYSICIANS at the time generally discouraged treatment of vision problems with corrective lenses. Instead, they favored and liberally prescribed therapeutic pharmaceutical remedies. In fact, spectacles were not commonly used in Europe for many years because of the sixteenth-century oculist and surgeon Georg Bartisch (who is often called the father of ophthalmology). In his widely-published writings, he opposed spectacles for vision correction, and lauded the use of eye powders and eye washes. His opinion was, "Man has two eyes — he needs not four." His words carried weight with those members of the medical community who wanted to debunk the wearing of spectacles as an unhealthy fad.[18]

There were, however, others who promoted their use. In seventeenth-century Spain, *Use of Spectacles for All Kinds of Sight* (1623) was written and published by Benito Daza de Valdes, a Jacobin friar. Spectacles were a stylish fashion accessory sported by the Spanish aristocracy: Legend has it that Marie Louise of Savoy, wife of King Philip V, arrived in Madrid with her 500 ladies-in-waiting all wearing identical tortoise-shell frame spectacles.[19]

The late 1700s marked the beginning of the European industrial revolution. The guilds' power waned in the onset of industrialization and lens manufacture improved greatly thanks to the introduction of cheaper production techniques made possible by technological advancements in optics and engineering. Craftsmen, who were no longer restricted by the guilds from travelling to other towns, shared their knowledge of a variety of time-honored techniques, improving the general education of all craftsmen. By the late 1700s, vendors of optical goods had a greater supply of higher-quality lenses to dispense.

BY THE HELP OF MY SPECTACLES

THE INDUSTRIAL REVOLUTION spread to the American colonies by the late eighteenth century. Many American spectaclemakers were silversmiths and opticians trained in the manufacture of microscopes and telescopes. Some were inspired by their British counterparts to aid clients in properly fitting lenses for their vision requirements. One noted source of inspiration was John Cuff, a Master of the Worshipful Company of Spectaclemakers, who served in King George III's court. He was renowned for his remarkable accuracy in manufacturing and fitting spectacles for his customers.[20]

But colonial physicians agreed with Bartisch's renunciation of the use of spectacles for vision correction, and most American colonists were more inclined to try British herbalist Nicholas Culpepper's folk remedies than to purchase spectacles. According to Culpepper, if the herb Eyebright (*euphrasia officinales*) "was but as much used as neglected, it would spoil the spectaclemaker's trade."[21]

Despite these trends, in 1783, James McAllister of Philadelphia reputedly opened the first optical shop devoted primarily to the measuring, fitting, and selling of spectacles. President Thomas Jefferson was one of McAllister's regular clients, sending him sketched specifications for custom-designed spring frame bifocals, and placing orders for magnifying goggles. McAllister is also attributed with being one of the first American producers of toric lenses which he reputedly made for another regular client, C.E. Goodrich.[22]

Benjamin Franklin, though frequently miscredited with the invention of bifocals, was the most famous of several people who designed a bicentric lens system. While serving as the American Ambassador to France, Franklin wrote a letter in August 1784, in which he declared that

toric lens: a lens which has curves at right angles to each other. it has no focal point, but it does have focal lines.

bicentric lens: a lens in which the upper portion focuses on distant objects while the lower portion focuses on near objects.

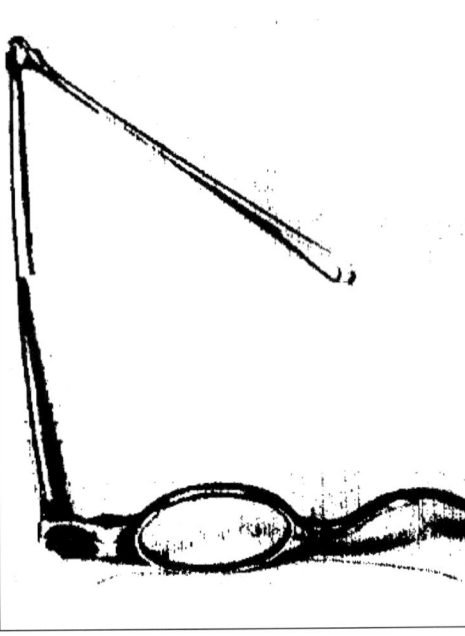

Thomas Jefferson gave optician James McAllister detailed specifications for the design of his spectacles.

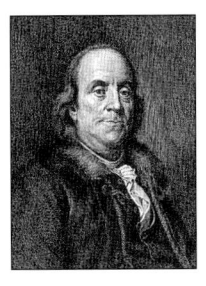

Benjamin Franklin, tired of carrying two pairs of spectacles, devised his own pair of bicentric bifocals.

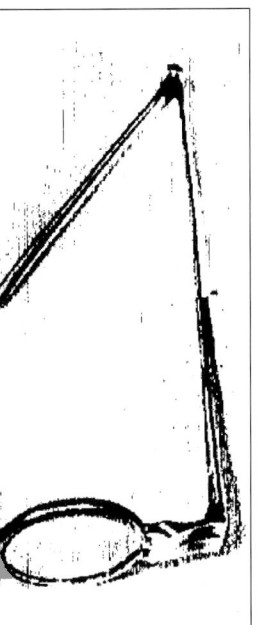

he was tired of carrying "two pairs of spectacles which I shifted occasionally, as in travelling I sometimes read and often wanted to regard the prospects. Finding this change troublesome and always sufficiently ready, I had the glasses cut and half of each kind associated in the same circle." By the next year, Franklin was even more elated with the results of his experiment. He wrote:[23]

> *By this means, as I wear my spectacles constantly, I have only to move my eyes up or down as I want to see distinctly far or near, the proper glasses always being ready. This I find more particularly convenient since my being in France, the glasses that serve me best at table to see what I eat, not being the best to see the faces of those on the other side of the table who speak to me; and when one's ears are not well accustomed to the sounds of a language, a sight of the movements in the features of him that speaks helps to explain; so that I understand French better by the help of my spectacles.[24]*

OCULISTS, OPHTHALMOLOGISTS, OPTICIANS, AND PEDDLERS

BY THE MID-NINETEENTH CENTURY, there were 3 common types of medical practitioner — household members who issued home remedies; physicians who prescribed a variety of treatments; and lay healers who practiced homeopathy, midwifery, and folk medicine. Physicians were fighting for a privileged status — for official recognition to set them apart from popular medicine's lay practitioners. They were also arguing among themselves as to whether they actually had any more effective therapies to offer. Specialization was blooming in the medical profession as science was discovering more about the sources of disease and human abnormalities.

Ophthalmology was one of those new specialties. Ophthalmologists were physicians who specialized in the diagnosis and treatment of eye diseases as well as the correction of vision malfunctions with eyedrops, eye powders, or corrective lenses. Karl Himley (reputedly the first professor on the subject) began teaching ophthalmology, in 1803, at a Göttingen university medical clinic.

Ophthalmology itself became recognized as a specialty about 50 years later when a number of hospitals dedicated to the treatment of eye diseases emerged in Great Britain and America. These facilities also trained medical professionals, who, by the American Civil War had grown considerably in number. In 1864, a group of these specialists met in New York City and formed the American Ophthalmological Society.[25]

Oculists — physicians who specialized in the treatment of eye, ear, nose, and throat problems — also examined eyes, prescribed formulas for corrective lenses, and sometimes even dispensed their own spectacle prescriptions.[26]

Outside the medical community, there were other professionals and tradesmen who provided vision care in America. Dispensing opticians supplied corrective lenses that were prescribed by an oculist or ophthalmologist. In contrast, refracting opticians measured patients' refractive condition. If a vision problem was detected, refracting opticians supplied patients with appropriate lenses. But if an eye disease or an uncorrectable abnormality was detected, these opticians referred their patients to ophthalmologists.[27]

Americans also purchased spectacles from local jewelers, watchmakers, and haberdashers. Some of the country's early refraction specialists were originally jewelers. Their skill in the manufacture of precision metal fittings made them ideal candidates for learning the techniques of eye measurement and lens fitting in the natural course of perfecting and selling their inventory.

There was a certain amount of animosity between these varied practitioners. Ophthalmologists and oculists felt that because the eye is part of the human body, the practice of ocular refraction fell within their area of expertise. Dispensing and refracting opticians were not medically-trained professionals and were, therefore, considered by the medical community to be nothing more than tradesmen.[28]

Despite the growing number of vision specialists, many urban and rural Americans continued to test their own vision by trying on spectacles selected from store and pharmacy display cases or from the lens peddler's cases until they found what seemed to be a correct pair. Fortunately for consumers, some shopkeepers discovered that

THE QUEST FOR BETTER VISION

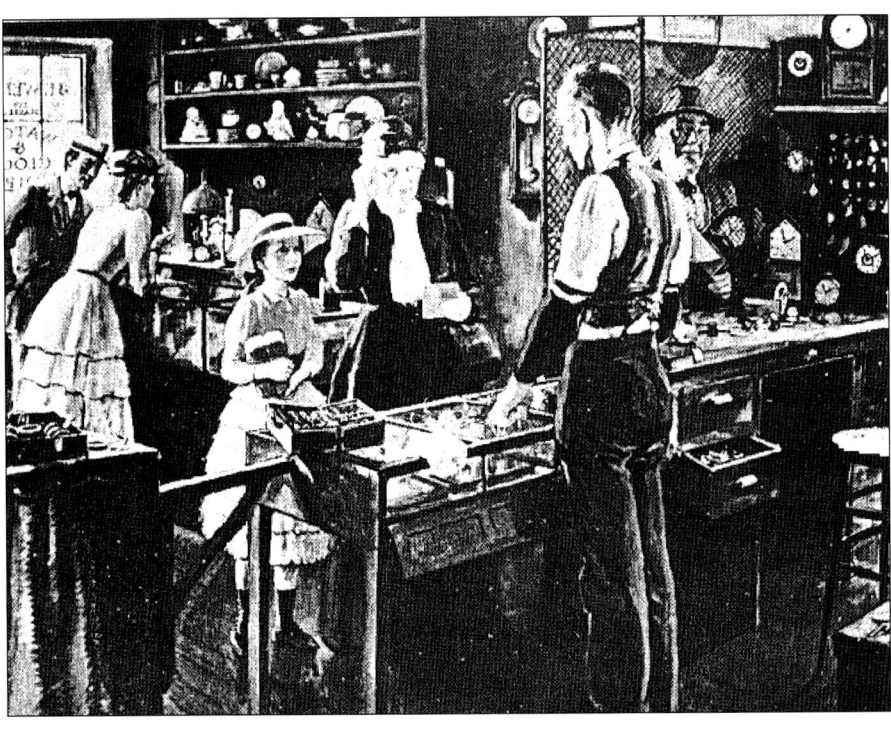

Spectacles were often sold in jewelry shops. Jewelers had the tools and materials to repair and manufacture eyewear frames.

by providing space for traveling opticians or by hiring resident refracting opticians they could increase their spectacle sales.[29]

American and Canadian lens peddlers travelled rugged frontier roads with their wares, selling spectacles to pioneering settlers who lived in remote areas of the continent. The peddler's trade continued well into the twentieth century, until optometric legislation was enacted nationwide in the 1930s and peddlers were no longer allowed to use ophthalmoscopes, optometers or any other vision testing devices. (Though many peddlers were honest, others were simply out to make a profit.)[30]

ophthalmoscope: an instrument used to examine the eye's interior.

optometer: an instrument used to measure the eye's refractive power by means of lenses or adjustable targets.

PIONEERING BETTER EQUIPMENT

IN 1847, BRITISH ASTRONOMER and lensmaker Charles Babbage invented the Babbage ophthalmoscope. The device provided its user with a clear view of a patient's retina via light reflected from an angled-mirror that had several small viewing holes drilled through its face. Though it wasn't until 4 years later when Hermann Ludwig Ferdinand von Helmholz, a Prussian physicist and physiologist, invented an improved ophthalmoscope and published his

ophthalmomter: an instrument used to measure the cornea's refractive power.

accommodation: the act of focusing the eye.

spherical lens: a lens with equal surface curvatures in all its meridians on both sides, bringing light to a pointed focus.

results, that the device became widely recognized as a valuable diagnostic tool. In 1866, von Helmholz developed an instrument which precisely measured the cornea's refracting power: recording the curvature of the central corneal area by determining the size of an image reflected by the cornea itself. Von Helmholz's ophthalmometer quickly proved to be a valuable instrument for both comparative studies in astigmatic cases and in general eye refraction examinations.[31]

Von Helmholz's major written work, *Physiological Optics* (1866) documented many centuries of observation and analysis of visual science. This work later served as one of theoretical optometry's foundations. He also formalized the still-accepted theory of color perception: that various combinations of 3 component colors — red, green, and blue — make up the entire visual mechanism that filters and perceives light in a full spectrum of hues. He also demonstrated the function of accommodation, and conceptualized the eye itself as a living, auto-focusing, optical instrument.[32]

During this time, it was widely believed that high-quality optical glass could not be produced in the United States. This was attributed to the differences in the available raw materials. Actually, it was just that no one with sufficient skills, knowledge, and equipment had attempted to produce optical glass until the mid-nineteenth century. Attitudes changed when Charles A. Spencer, a New York microscope maker, won the 1878 Paris Exposition's Gold Medal. He had successfully produced very high-quality optical glass for his instruments from American raw materials.[33]

By the 1880s, another manufacturer, the American Optical Company of Southbridge, Massachusetts, was also mass-producing its own spherical lens line created from domestic raw materials, instead of importing European goods. A new era in optical services, products, and manufacturing had finally taken root in America.[34]

During the nineteenth-century, instrumentation that accurately measured human vision was developed and produced. By the end of the century, there were numerous versions of optometers, refractometers, and trial cases marketed to the growing number of eye treatment specialists.

THE QUEST FOR BETTER VISION

15

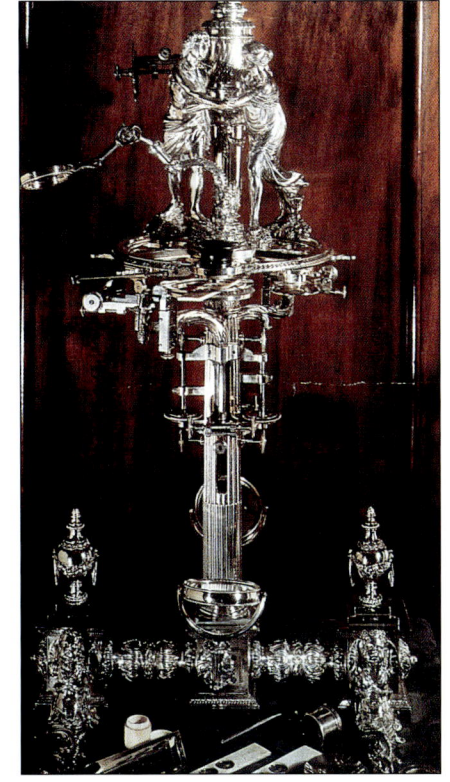

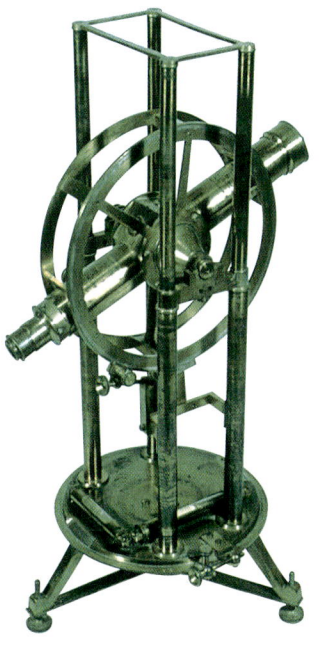

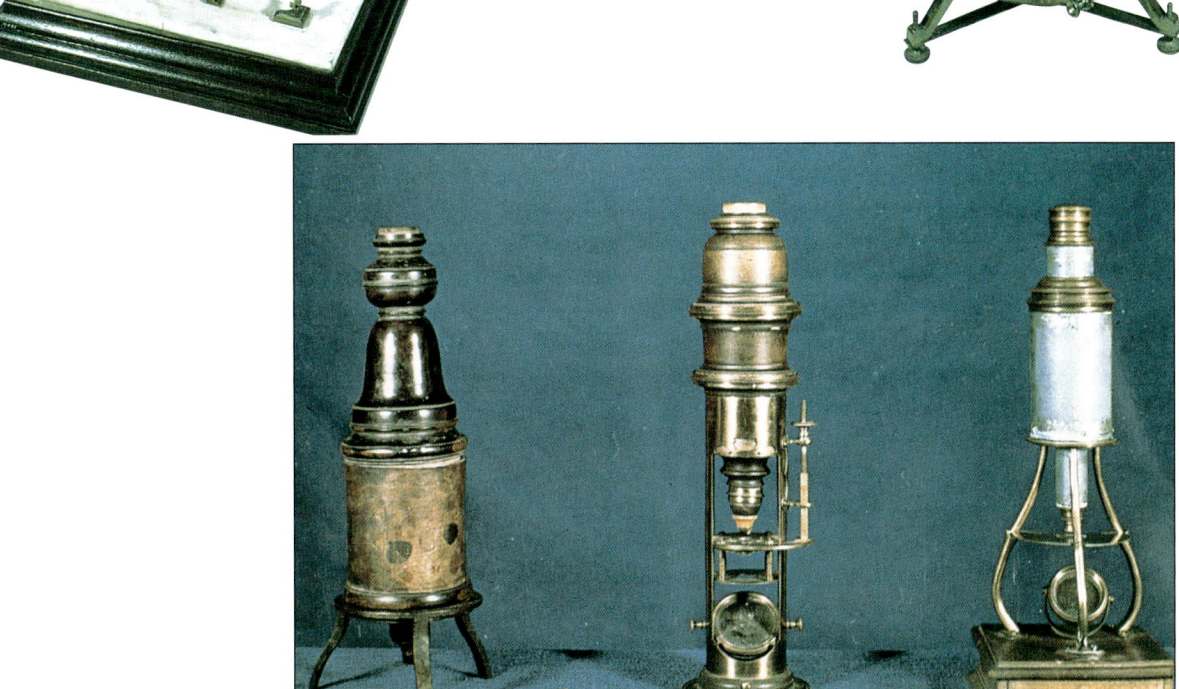

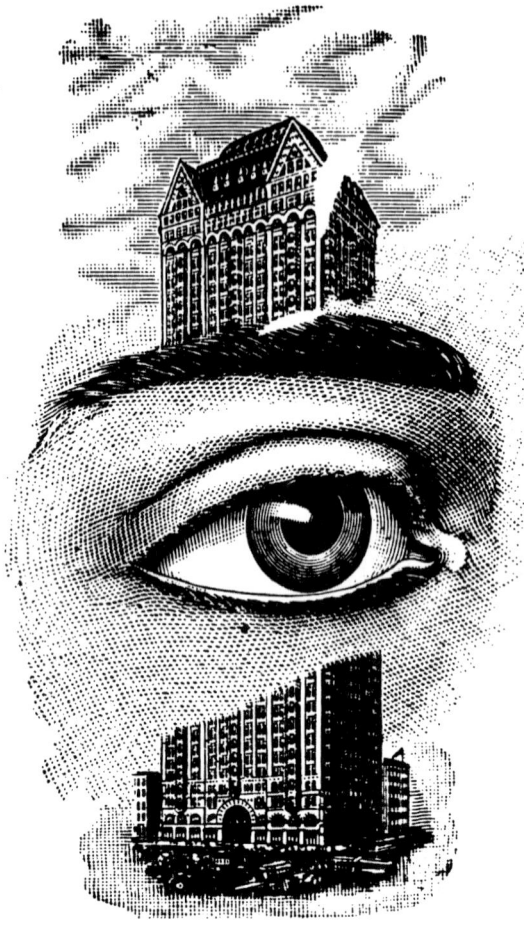

CHAPTER 2

The LARGEST *and* BEST EQUIPPED *in the* WORLD

NORTHERN ILLINOIS COLLEGE
OF OPHTHALMOLOGY & OTOLOGY

AMERICA INDUSTRIALIZES

As the American population grew so did the number of medical specialists treating vision-related problems.

THE VICTORIAN ERA had transformed both Europe and America. Nineteenth-century technological advancements, increased manufacturing, and social reform turned predominantly agrarian nations into industrial giants in less than half a century. In America, midwestern cities like Chicago and St. Louis grew out of a need to link the raw materials of the west with the manufacturing and distribution centers of the east. Wagon train trails, stretching from the Atlantic to the Pacific, gave way to railroad tracks. Horse-drawn railroad trains

17

(like the early B&O Railroad) were eventually replaced by steam-powered locomotives and freight cars. By the 1860s, all routes led to Chicago. In less than 50 years, the city had grown from a small military outpost into a thriving industrial metropolis. In 1871, the Great Fire incinerated 3.5 square miles of the city in 16 hours, but less than a year later, the city rose from the ashes and, once again, took its place as the American Heartland's commercial and industrial hub.[1]

During this same time, passenger trains imported America's most vital commodity: people. They travelled by coach and train from neighboring farm towns and the bayous of the South. They sailed from from impoverished or politically-oppressed communities overseas, and worked for their passage to the nation's interior. They came from everywhere; and they all hoped to latch onto a corner of the prospering American Dream. The nation's cities, including Chicago, grew at a staggering rate.

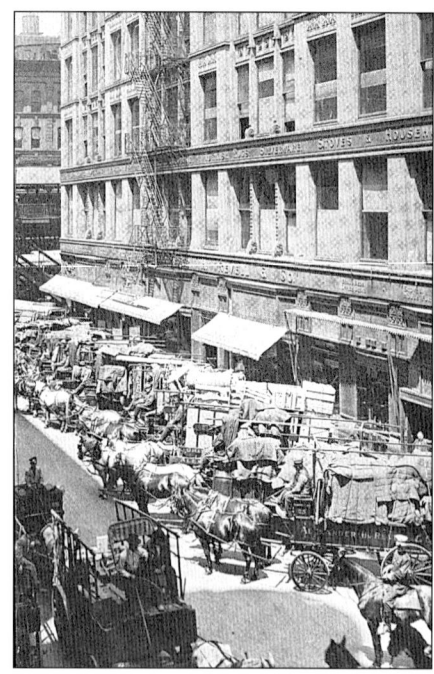

From the ashes of the Great Fire in 1871, Chicago built a major metropolis in America's heartland.

At the same time advancements in the printing process made books, magazines, and newspapers even cheaper to produce. An increasingly literate public demanded as much information as could be typeset and printed. There were more leisure hours made available to read all this information because of another new invention: the electric light bulb. And skilled production jobs required closer, more detailed work than agricultural labor had demanded. Limited or faulty vision became a much greater liability, and made the demand for vision care far more pressing.

People were living longer. Federal and state public-health agencies were improving their knowledge and treatment of the public's health, beginning with improvements in sanitation. These programs eventually extending to include personal hygiene, health education, and the establishment of public health dispensaries for the care of poor patients who could not afford adequate medical care. But the medical community fought against this intrusion into their market and eventually quashed it: after all, these were the same people who filled private practices and privately-owned hospitals. They refined their specializations and campaigned for strict legislation which would guaranty their total authority over the medical profession.[2]

But the profession that would become optometry was growing, independent of the medical profession's control. Among the practitioners and educators, leaders were emerging; and advances in technology were booming. The U.S. Patent office recorded 44 new patents for optometers and refractometers alone between 1874 and 1899.[2]

refractometer: similar to an optometer, this instrument measured the eye's refractive power.

TEACHING PRACTICAL SCIENTIFIC METHODS OF FITTING SPECTACLES

IN 1879, JUST AS CHICAGO began its greatest expansion period, James Burton McFatrich arrived from Lena, Illinois. The son of a small town doctor, McFatrich had earned his Master of Science degree at Upper Iowa University, and had moved to Chicago to further his education.[3]

He attended 2 Chicago medical schools — Hahnemann Medical College, and Bennett College of Medicine and Surgery. Bennett College's ophthalmology and otology department was chaired by Dr. Henry Olin whose successful career included an extensive practice, important discoveries about the ear's physiology, and new operative procedures for clearing nasal duct obstructions. In 1872, Olin founded the Chicago College of Ophthalmology and Otology which tutored medical students and professionals in post-graduate eye and ear care as well as refraction.[4]

otology: a medical specialty dedicated to the treatment and diagnosis of diseases or dysfunctions of the ear.

Olin's college outgrew its Madison Street medical office space in 1878, so Olin moved into a larger classroom on State Street and incorporated the institution. By the late 1890s, the faculty had grown to include 5 instructors.[5]

There were other optically-oriented post-graduate medical schools in the Chicago area: the McCormick Optical College, the Johnston Optical Institute, and The Chicago Ophthalmic College which had its own hospital and dispensary. Nationwide, 60 independent schools had emerged to train students in this new specialty.[6]

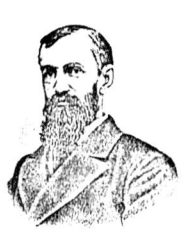

Dr. Henry Olin established the Chicago College of Ophthalmology and Otology to instruct medical practitioners in both specialities.

AN ECLIPSE IN THE OPTICAL WORLD

IN 1887, DR. OLIN invited Dr. James McFatrich, who had just completed a 2-year Cook County Hospital internship, to become a full partner in his rapidly expanding enterprise. Dr. McFatrich quickly established a bustling ophthalmological practice. He also accepted a teaching position at Bennett College, and joined Dr. Olin's faculty. When Olin retired in 1889 for health reasons, McFatrich took over both the practice and the school's management. Following Olin's death in 1891, Dr. McFatrich assumed complete control of the school. He changed the institution's name to Northern Illinois College of Ophthalmology and Otology (NICOO), and relocated the school to the new 20-story Masonic Temple Building at the corner of State and Randolph Streets.[7]

James' brother, George Wilbur McFatrich, completed his training at Bennett College and became a Cook County Hospital house physician in 1892. Eighteen months later, he was appointed to be the hospital's attending surgeon and oculist. He was then elected Professor of Ophthalmology and Otology at Bennett College. George also joined the NICOO staff and, in 1896, the McFatrich brothers incorporated the school with themselves and their younger sister, Mary, as its sole stockholders and corporate officers.[8]

NICOO's letterhead proudly proclaimed: "Practical Scientific Methods of Fitting Spectacles and Eyeglasses Taught by a Capable Faculty" and "Largest and Best Equipped in the World. Incorporated Under Laws of State of Illinois."[9]

And their trade journal advertisements prominently displayed the Masonic Temple Building, so prospective students would associate the towering skyscraper with the prominence of both the school and the rising profession it taught.[10]

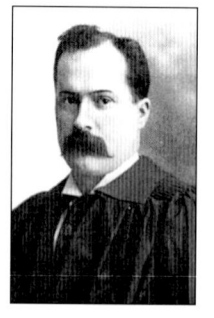

Dr. James McFatrich not only made his school the nation's largest institution dedicated to the teaching of refraction, he also made his eyedrop company a household word.

FACING PAGE: George McFatrich launched an aggressive advertising campaign proudly proclaiming NICOO as the largest and best equipped in the world.

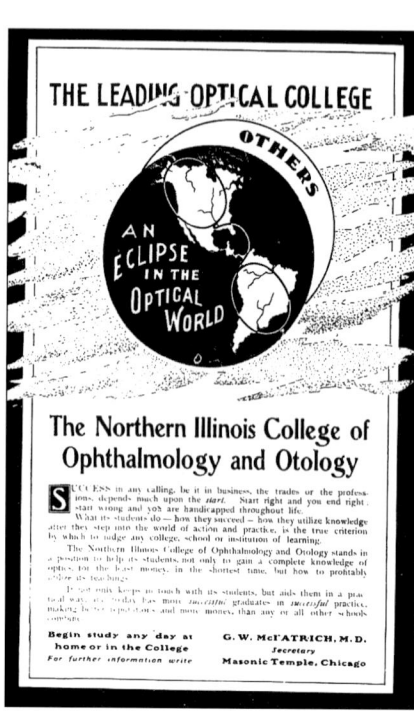

Eclipse in the Optical World was one of many ads used to promote the Northern Illinois College of Ophthalmology and Otology.

THE LARGEST AND
BEST EQUIPPED
IN THE WORLD

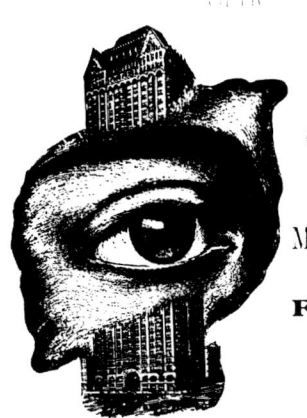

Northern Illinois College of Ophthalmology and Otology.

Masonic Temple, Chicago.

Full Course in Optics with all privileges

$25.00

FACULTY:
JAMES BURTON McFATRICH, M. S., M. D. — Professor of the Principles of Ophthalmology and Otology.
GEORGE WILBUR McFATRICH, M. D. — Professor of Clinical Ophthalmology and Otology.
GEORGE A. ROGERS. — Professor of Optometry.
H S TYNER, A. M., M. D. — Professor of Anatomy and Physiology of Eye and Brain.
C. PORTER JOHNSON, L. B., LL.D. — Professor of Optical Jurisprudence.
J. KITTREDGE WHEELER, D. D. — Professor of Psychology.
H. F. BENNETT, M. D. — Professor of Microscopy and Histology.
E. J. TROWBRIDGE, M. D. — Professor of Optics.
HAROLD E. THOMAS, O. D. — Instructor on Anatomy and Refraction.

The evolution of the optician, from what he has been to what he is, and from what he is to what he will become, is mainly a question of

EDUCATION.

The influences of association, organization, co-operation and legislation can be of no practical value or advantage to him until he has been grounded in optics by good, hard, practical schooling at a first class optical training school. That should be his foundation.

THE NORTHERN ILLINOIS COLLEGE is not only the most thoroughly equipped, best at practical optical school in America, but these thin a great outlay. Its running expenses, includin month are greater than the annual expenses of mo competitors.

ITS LARGER ADVANTA

The fact that it is a school on a large scale is to its students. They have associates, form acquai study together and finally constitute a vast alumni. and fire of discussion and debate due to numbers, principle with a clearness *that individual study* cou

Educate yourself first and then join hands general advancement.

Address all inquiries to

GEO. W. McFATRICH, M. D., Sec'y
No. 1015 MASONIC TE

NORTHERN ILLINOIS COLLEGE
OF
Ophthalmology AND Otology

A PRACTICAL TRAINING SCHOOL FOR OPTICIANS.

Masonic Temple,   Chicago.

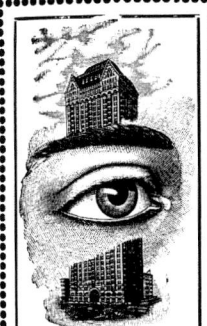

THE Matriculation Fee, $25.00, entitles you to the certificate, "Fellow in Optics," which is a **Life** Scholarship and admits you to any and all courses at any and all times.

Correspondence and Attendance Courses.

The "McFatrich Eye" (patented 1902) with pamphlet, $2.00
Lenses for the "Eye"   :   :   :   1.00

If you have a trial case you will not need the lenses. A discount on the "Eye" wi be allowed students of this college.

We confer upon all graduates the degree, "Doctor of Optics," and as an inducement to continued study and advanced work, the degrees, "Bachelor of Ophthalmology," "Master of Ophthalmology," and "Doctor of Ophthalmology."

If you have not received a copy of our 1903 Announcement, write for it.

GEO. W. McFATRICH, M. D., SECRETARY.

The McFatriches established another enterprise in 1897: the Murine Eye Remedy Company. James McFatrich had developed a muriate of berberine-based eyedrop formula which he used extensively in his own practice. Otis F. Hall, a Spokane, Washington banker, was so impressed with the product that he persuaded McFatrich to market Murine nationwide and became his business partner.[11]

With the success of this new venture, James McFatrich turned over much of the school's management to his brother George: he maintained his medical practice, managed the Murine Eye Remedy Company, and became closely involved with masonic and political activities.

James McFatrich also contributed many articles to professional journals, campaigning the need for more optical education. "The condition of the optical business — we use this term in contradistinction to that of the optical profession — is deplorable," he wrote in a 1902 *Optical Journal* article. "No one who does not come into intimate contact with it can have the faintest idea of the ignorance that pervades the calling. Men, who as jewelers or traveling spectacle peddlers, have engaged in the business for years. In thousands of cases they have no knowledge whatever of the science of optics. … We have met 'opticians,' incredible as it may appear, who did not know what a focus was. But they can sell spectacles." His

Northern Illinois College of Ophthalmology and Otology trained both medical and non-medical students in the precise science of refraction.

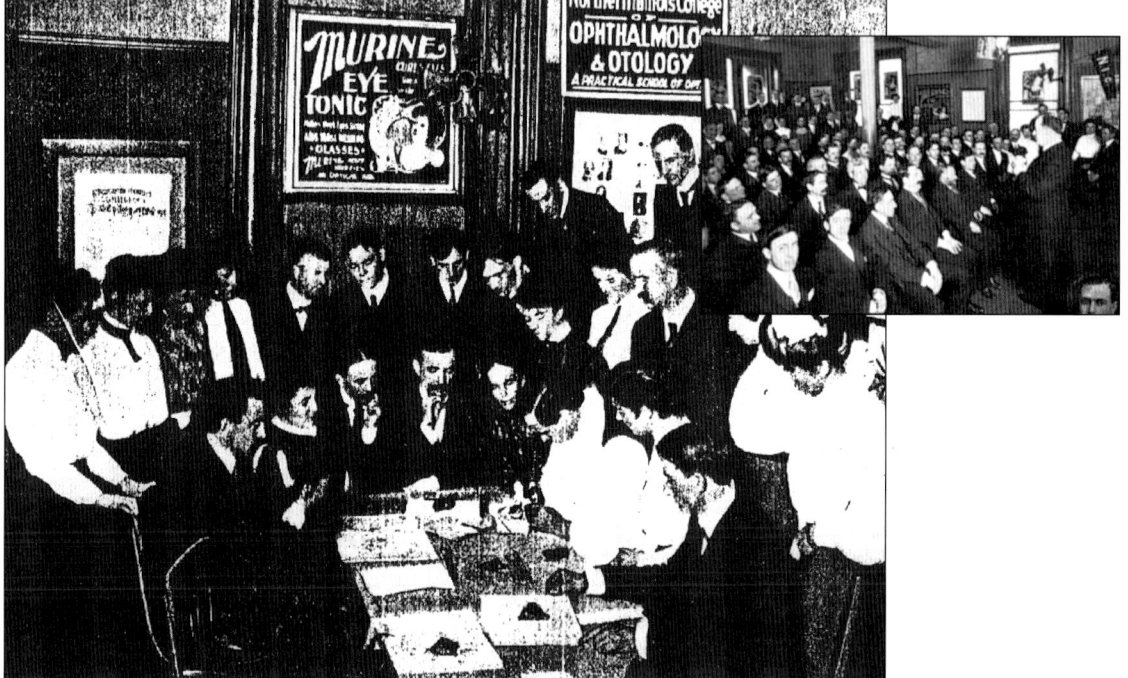

observations were correct: at that time, many people were still purchasing corrective eyewear from untrained vendors, without the benefit of an examination.[12]

His solution to this crisis was to redouble his efforts to promote education. "Education pays," he concluded, "and is a means of safety to the practitioner, for the optician is as liable in damages for his mistakes as the physician is; and the only reason that he has not been held more strictly accountable for serious blunders is because people have not valued the eye and its treatment as they are rapidly coming to value it." Public demand for better quality health care in the United States coupled with the need for more properly-trained caregivers was growing as the nation's population increased. But generally, there was still little regard for improved vision care.[13]

Under George McFatrich's administration, NICOO changed both its admission policies and its scope. Since its establishment, the school had restricted its student body to post-graduate medical students and doctors — primarily from Bennett College, and Cook County Hospital. George McFatrich amended the school's charter, in 1898, to include the admission of non-medical candidates who already had some practical experience and knowledge: the majority were jewelers, refracting and dispensing opticians. He discontinued the otology courses (although he kept the subject in the school's title). To deter conflict with the medical community, McFatrich noted in the school's 1909 catalog: "The college does not confer any right whatever upon the graduate to practice medicine, but trains them to accurately correct errors of refraction by fitting glasses properly, to practice as an optician with credit to themselves and to the college." Even so, the prospect of starting a respectable professional career for an investment of $25 in tuition and an additional $15-65 in lens inventory plus office space was very alluring to any ambitious, entrepreneurial person.[14]

THE LARGEST AND BEST EQUIPPED IN THE WORLD

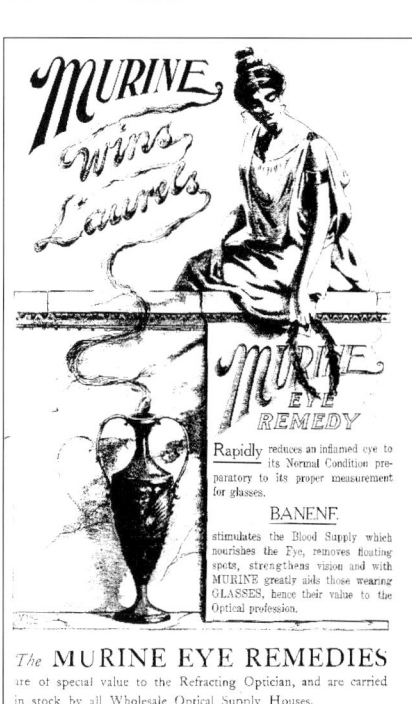

Murine Eyedrops were the most famous of the many eye care products developed and manufactured by the Drs. McFatrich and their partner Otis Hall.

refraction: the bending of light as it travels between an object and the eye. Also refers to the act of measuring the eye's refractive power.

trial case: a case containing concave, convex, and spherical lenses, along with cylinders, prisms and other testing devices.

astigmatism: a condition where there are 2 focal lines instead of a single focal point.

retinoscopy: the measurement of the eye's refractive condition.

Prior to this, only a couple of institutions accepted non-medical students. The Spencer Optical Institute, operated by The Spencer Optical Manufacturing Company, offered a 2-week ocular refraction training course. For $25 the institute trained students in basic refraction and use of the Audemaire Trial Case (the company's own product). And the King Optical Company of Cleveland, Ohio offered a similar week-long course to promote their Elite Test Case.[15]

To meet the demands of a larger student body, George McFatrich added more teaching staff and courses. He wrote a number of the college's standard texts himself, covering studies of astigmatism, retinoscopy, ophthalmology, and muscular imbalance. His articles on topics such as subjective and objective testing regularly appeared in *The Optical Journal*. He also introduced a series of week-long postgraduate seminars aimed at updating practitioners on the latest discoveries and developments in their field.[16]

McFatrich then launched another major recruitment campaign. In 1899, ads placed in *The Optical Journal* and other publications proudly listed the school's experienced faculty, which by that time, included Drs. James B. and George W. McFatrich, Professors of Ophthalmology and Clinical Ophthalmology; Dr. Henry S. Tucker, Professor of Neurology; C. Porter Johnson, Professor of Medical Jurisprudence; Rev. J. Kittredge Wheeler, Professor of Psychology; and Dr. H.F. Bennett, Professor of Optics.[17]

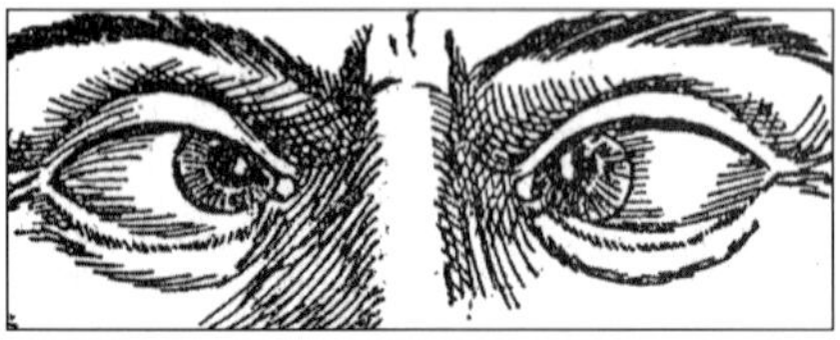

Rev. Wheeler was replaced, in 1905, by Dr. Chalmers Prentice, who became the school's Professor of Latent Brain Strain. Prentice was a well-known author of the time who had written a book on the therapeutic value of lenses entitled *The Eye in Its Relation to Health*.[18]

Later, Dr. Tucker was promoted to Professor of Physiology of the Eye and Brain; and the former principal of the Chicago Post-Graduate Optical College, Dr. George A. Rogers was hired to teach the new science of - optometry.[19]

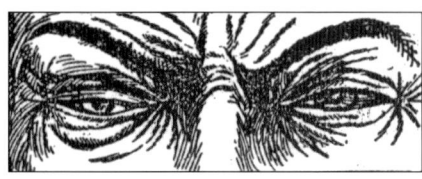

The new sport of Ping-pong caused concern among early 1900s eye specialists. It was feared that viewers might become victims of "ping pong squint" if they focussed too intently on the ball.

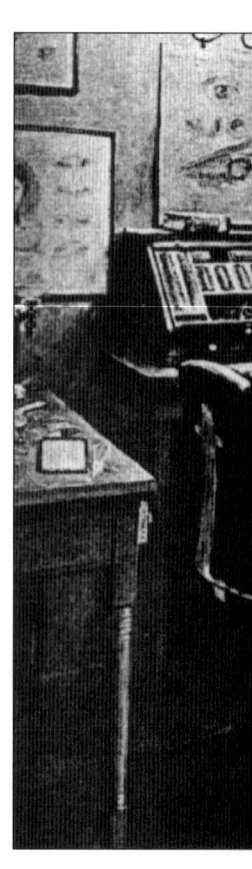

Many early practitioners examined patients eyes in space rented inside jewelry shops and department stores.

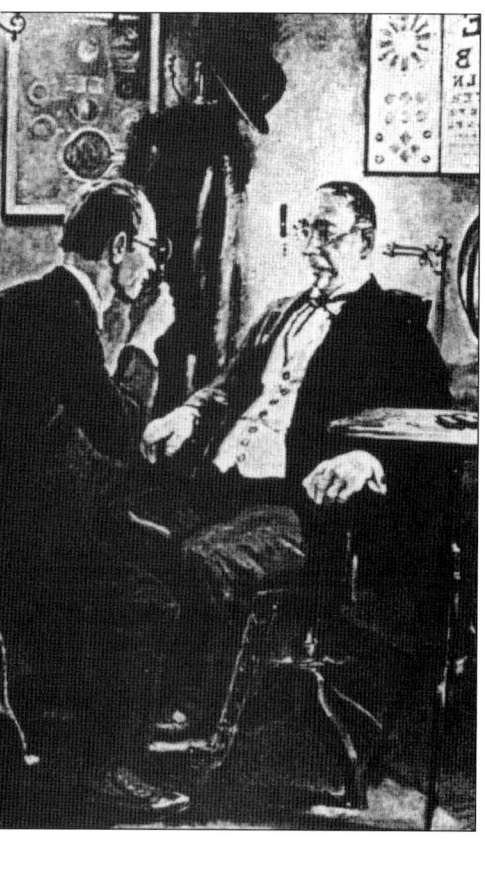

During the late 1890s and early 1900s, the former Lieutenant Governor of Illinois, Lawrence Y. Sherman, taught optical jurisprudence. Basic legal training introduced students to the parameters of their professional practice and its application according to the various states' licensing requirements.[20]

Public sentiment about spectacles shifted to the positive end of the spectrum when, in 1902, Theodore Roosevelt succeeded William McKinley as President of the United States. Generally, the public had believed only weak or sickly people wore spectacles. But when illustrations appeared in daily newspapers nationwide depicting a spectacle-wearing Roosevelt charging up Cuba's San Juan Hill with his Rough Riders during the 1898 Spanish-American War, the myth was debunked. But Roosevelt wasn't the only President to sport oxford frames, Calvin Coolidge also wore them when he was in the White House.

THE LARGEST AND BEST EQUIPPED IN THE WORLD

oxford frames: pince-nez attached by a piece of cord or ribbon to the wearer's clothing so they dangled close at hand when not in use.

EVERY ARTISAN IS PRIVILEGED TO PUT HIS OWN PRICE UPON HIS TIME AND SKILL

WHILE THE MCFATRICH brothers were establishing their school, comprehensive nationwide regulation of the health care professions was well under way: guidelines for practice and the scopes of medical specialties and related health professions were being legally defined.[21]

The American Medical Association (AMA) was tightening its reign on who could — or could not — treat patients and charge a fee for professional services. They had already discouraged their own ranks from becoming "company doctors" — salaried physicians employed by in-

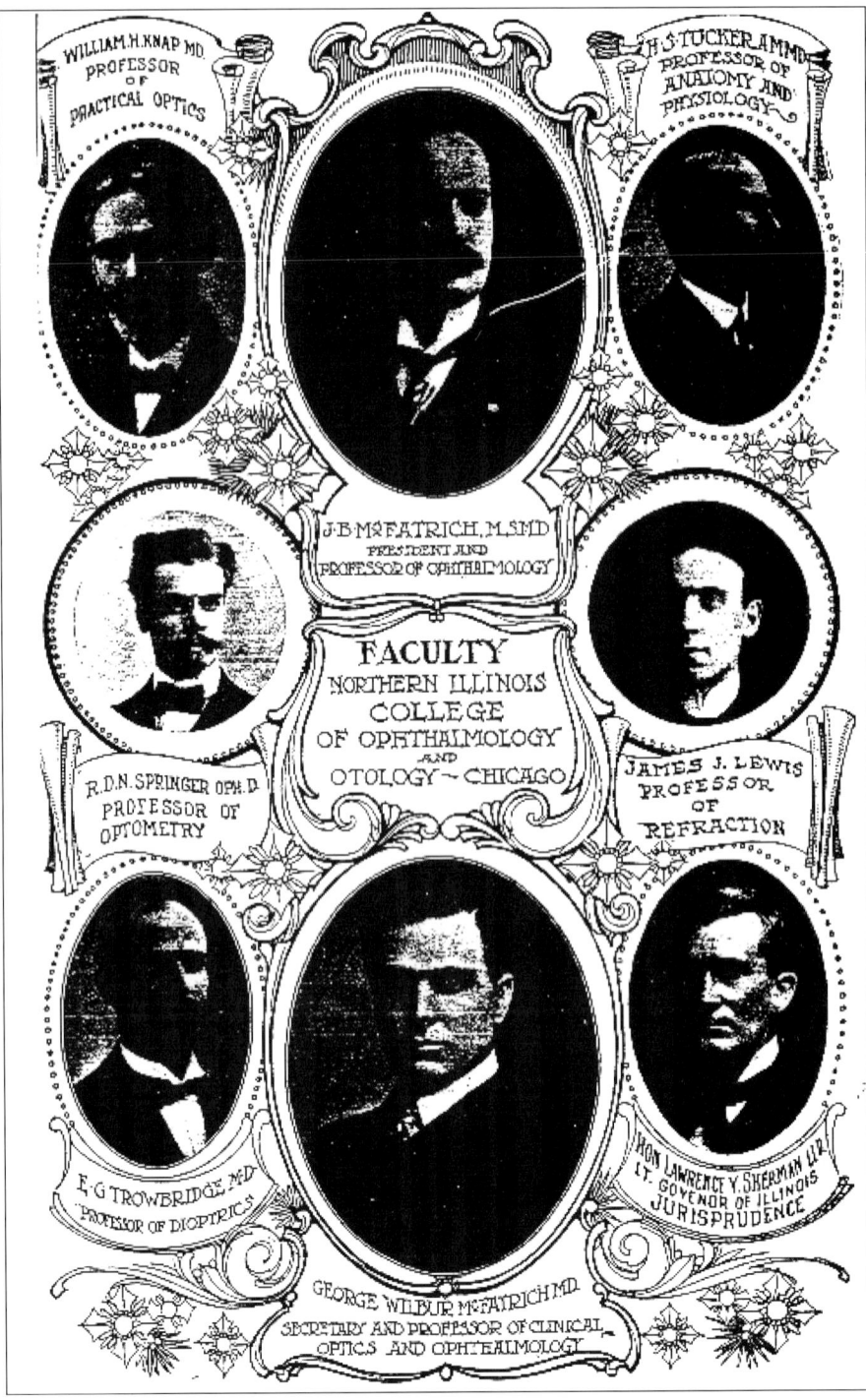

The faculty at Northern Illinois College of Optometry not only instructed students in the art of refraction, but also prepared students to understand the legal aspects of their profession and patient psychology.

dustry to keep employees healthy at no cost to the employees and with no procedure-based charges. They had also effectively lobbied against physicians providing services for fraternal and masonic organizations who would, in turn, offer prepaid, flat-fee medical care for their members. Much like today's HMOs (health maintenance organizations), organizers hoped to reduce rising health care costs by packaging customized payment plans that were beneficial to both the participating physicians and patients.[22]

Charles F. Prentice of New York (no relation to Dr. Chalmers Prentice) is credited with being the first American optician to charge an examination fee ($3 for a consultation), and to derive his income from both diagnostic and dispensing sources. Despite his many achievements, including research into the cause and treatment of astigmatism, Prentice's greatest contribution to the profession was his response to a letter. The controversy began in 1892, when Manhattan-based physician Dr. Henry D. Noyes wrote Prentice a thank-you letter for a patient referral. Noyes finished his genial correspondence by saying:[23]

> *I consider the matter to be serious, not because a competition is set up, but because an injustice is done to the public by the fact that in charging a fee you assume that you have the qualifications which entitle you to a fee for advice. To this I strenuously object and I beg call your attention to the subject most seriously and yet kindly.*[24]

Prentice's response to this reprimand was simple:

> *All my patrons are distinctly given to understand that I am not a physician, that I do not prescribe medicine, or give advice in a medical sense; but that the fee is intended to cover my scientifically conducted mechanical services, precisely in the same manner that a designer charges for his services in preparing his plans and specifications. In this sense every artisan is privileged to put his own price upon his time and skill… Besides, if I did not charge a fee for services rendered, I should be obliged to exact an extortionate price for the glasses, which is the method generally practiced by the charlatan.*[25]

This landmark exchange and an ensuing volley of correspondence with another physician, Dr. D.B. St. John Roosa, ended in Roosa's appeal to the New York County Medical Society for the ejection of members who referred patients to opticians for eyewear fitting.[26]

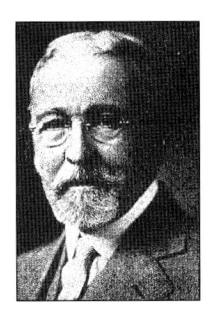

THE LARGEST AND BEST EQUIPPED IN THE WORLD

27

Charles F. Prentice stood firmly on his belief that his advice was worth a consultation fee, proclaiming, "every artisan is privileged to put his own price upon his time and skill."

Forced by the medical community's stand, dispensing opticians sided against refracting opticians as lobbying for New York legislation accelerated. To protect their rights, Prentice, along with Dr. Andrew J. Cross and other New York practitioners (including some refracting opticians) organized a professional group in 1896. They dedicated themselves to the "legalization" of optometry and called the organization The Optical Society of the State of New York.[27]

The struggle that followed in the state legislatures and the courts was quite similar to concurrent cases instigated by the AMA against laboratory technicians, midwives, and anesthetists.[28]

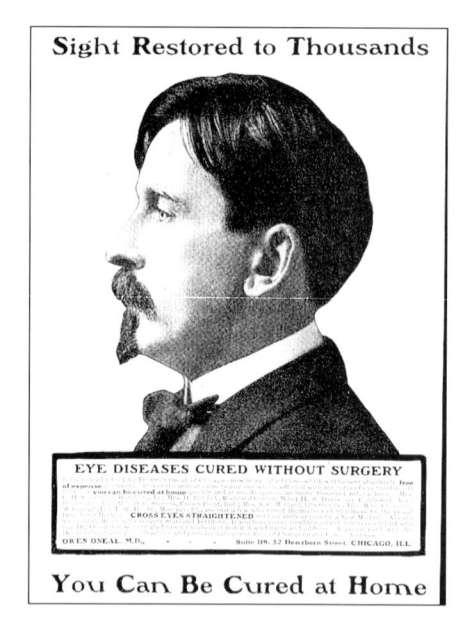

Early opticians offered the public a non-surgical alternative to their vision problems.

THE EMPLOYMENT OF SUBJECTIVE AND OBJECTIVE MECHANICAL MEANS

MORE REFRACTING OPTICIANS and oculists followed Prentice and Cross' examples nationwide. They lobbied state legislatures for the establishment of optometric educational and professional standards. In 1901, the state of Minnesota passed the nation's first laws regulating optometric practice, licensing and education.

In 1898, Great Britain's Worshipful Company of Spectaclemakers had instituted periodic re-certification examinations for practicing refractionists. Members of the British Optical Association (founded in 1895) were also periodically re-examined and re-certified. And The Institute of Ophthalmic Opticians (an organization founded in 1905, which primarily served as a protective body for its members) required all applicants to be licensed by either of its predecessor organizations. But none of the associations outside of the United States had yet adopted the term "optometry" in reference to their profession.[29]

The Minnesota law defined optometry as: "the employment of subjective and objective mechanical means to determine the accommodative and refractive states of the eye and the scope of its functions in general." A state-regulated examining board was established to test and license practicing optometrists. The law exempted ophthalmologists and non-prescriptive eyewear retailers — dispensing opticians, shopkeepers, and lens peddlers who did not attempt to use trial cases, ophthalmometers, and optometers in their marketing efforts — from regulation.[30]

The minimum 2000 hours of coursework required for licensing in Minnesota included:

125 hours	Ocular anatomy
125 hours	Ocular pathology
150 hours	General anatomy
100 hours	General physiology
150 hours	General mathematics
100 hours	General physics
100 hours	General optics
300 hours	Theoretical optics
100 hours	Practical optics
250 hours	Theoretical optometry
200 hours	Practical optometry
50 hours	Hygiene
50 hours	Psychology
100 hours	Optical laboratory
100 hours	Clinical work [31]

Many schools, including NICOO, continued to offer prospective students the option of completing 20 percent of their course work by correspondence rather than actual attendance despite the new requirements. But it limited the states in which graduates could practice.[32]

This was a radical increase in course hours over the short refraction courses most schools offered — including NICOO. Medical and dental schools faced similar new regulations. As state legislatures nationwide adopted laws over the next 24 years, remaining educational institutions, with the aid of the newly-established professional associations, eagerly reorganized their curricula.

All of the health care professions — including medicine, dentistry, and optometry — were defining their roles at this time. And although the early 1900s brought increased regulation to the professions, there were still many underqualified practitioners competing with highly-skilled professionals. But additional external recognition in the shape of state legislation, examination, and licensing was finally being established nationwide. Through professional associations, internal regulation of education and practice rose to a level that had not been reached since the time of the medieval guilds.

In 1910, the AMA's Council on Medical Education commissioned the Carnegie Foundation for the Advancement of Teaching to review the state of North American medical schools. Their report, *Medical Education in the United States and Canada* written by Alexander Flexner, harshly criticized the quality of American medical education; and stated that the medical professions were overcrowded with poorly-trained physicians. (This was not a blow to the professions, but rather an added weapon for those who sought reform.) Within a decade, the number of American medical schools declined from 162, in 1906, to 85, in 1920, as the professions refined their status.[33]

Even before legislation was enforced, there were several independent American and Canadian optometry schools whose courses contained more study hours in both theoretical and practical ocular refraction than could be found at any university-based medical college. But by 1914, more state licensing boards patterned themselves after Minnesota, and soon after, all schools required students to complete 2 years of high school study with special concentration on science courses prior to admission; and 2 years of attendance courses at an accredited optometry school before licensing.[34]

Naturally, the law of attrition came into play. Many small, independent schools did not survive this shakedown: by 1922, only 30 out of the 60 independent American optometry schools remained in operation. But NICOO complied with the states' mandates and successfully made the admission and curriculum transitions.[35]

During the late 1890s, NICOO had the distinguished lecturer and optometrist Dr. Andrew Jay Cross on its faculty. Dr. Cross had pioneered critical research in the development of monocentric bifocal lenses and dynamic skiametry.[36]

In addition to founding the Optical Society of the State of New York (OSSNY), Dr. Cross had become a powerful lobbyist for the optometric profession on the national level. In 1898, he had been elected president of OSSNY, and, two years later, Cross became the first optometrist elected president of the American Association of Opticians, a professional organization that was born from the writings of a publisher.[37]

Founder of *The Optical Journal and Review of Optometry*, Frederick Boger wrote, in 1895, that "an American association covering the whole country is what is needed, and the men to run it should step forward and unite." On October 10th, 1898, they did. A meeting took place at the Broadway Central Hotel in New York: the first gathering of charter members in the American Association of Opticians. In attendance were 150 of the 183 members — refracting and dispensing opticians, optical manufacturers, suppliers, importers and other interested parties. Like the AMA (which was founded with the same small membership and strong desire to attain professional stature in 1848) the association sought legislation and educational standardization for its national membership.[38]

By the 1906 convention, association membership had grown by over 900 percent. In a pre-convention mailing, the membership figures and the list of state affiliations told the story:

> We have organized under auspices of the National body, seven state societies, affiliated twelve states and added nearly eight hundred new members, more than have been enrolled during the previous six years of the organization.[39]

Outside the convention and the association, use of the title of "doctor" in relation to the optometric profession was being hotly debated. The AMA adopted a resolution to instigate prosecution of non-medical refractionists, optometrists, and both types of opticians. The AMA lobbied for a Supreme Court decision on the interpretation the practice of optometry as a violation of the medical practice. But optometrists were also seeking nationwide legal recognition, and by this time, 24 states had already passed laws

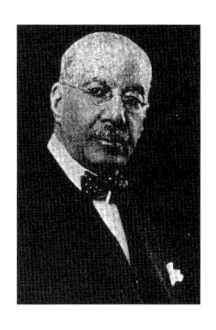

refractionists: specialists who measured the eye's refractive power.

Andrew J. Cross was one of optometry's early pioneers, lobbying for regulated licensing and educational requirements throughout the nation.

affirming optometry's professional status.⁴⁰ The American Association of Opticians responded to the AMA's attacks by establishing a public education committee, and developing a uniform state-examination syllabus.⁴¹

Reorganization and re-delegation of special committees seemed to occur regularly within the association during those years, refining its intentions and purposes to better suit the needs of a burgeoning profession. By 1912, the association's Education Committee's curriculum recommendations were adopted. Five levels of concentration were outlined which more closely resembled the Minnesota law. By raising educational requirements and encouraging adoption of higher standards by all state boards, the committee hoped to further establish the profession's standing in the eyes of the federal government and the public.⁴²

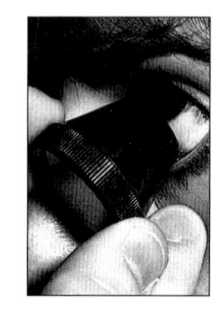

Three years later, the National Organization of State Boards of Examiners in Optometry did adopt those recommendations, and added that 75 percent was the minimum passing score on written examinations; that the standard of clinic work at optometric schools had to be elevated as high as possible; and that optometric schools had to require applicants to complete at least two years of high-school education. The association finally voted, at the 1919 convention, to change its name to the American Optometric Association (AOA) in recognition of the profession they now strongly represented.⁴³

The Thorington Retinoscope (1902) was just the beginning of an extensive list of optometric equipment and optical advancements made between 1900 and 1920. Until this time, there was no standard optometric examination procedure. Practitioners measured patients' visual function as they saw fit. But standardization began in 1917, when an Ohio State University optometry professor, Dr. Charles Sheard, published his 18-point testing technique entitled *Dynamic Ocular Tests*. This series of analytic procedures — later amended to 21 points — vastly improved practitioners' analytic and diagnostic procedures. Even the faintest vision dysfunctions could be detected and corrected with increased accuracy and reliability. These pro-

During the early part of the century, new instrumentation developments improved the accuracy of optometric examinations. Equipment like the campimeter, perimeter, gonioscope (pictured above), keratometer, and visual acuity apparatus made education even more critical to the profession. Continuing education classes helped working practitioners upgrade their skills.

retinoscope: an instrument used to objectively measure the eye's refractive condition.

cedures became the basis for modern optometry's foundations as the century progressed.[44]

FELLOWS IN OPTICS

PRIOR TO THE 1908 PASSAGE of the State of Illinois' optometric legislation, NICOO conferred a Doctor of Optics degree on students who completed a 4-week attendance course or a 6-week correspondence course. The full $25 tuition, paid in advance, entitled each student to become a "'Fellow in Optics' which is a Life Scholarship." For an additional $2, students received the "McFatrich Eye" model; and for another $1, they could purchase a trial case. The entire fee was equivalent to a skilled laborer's monthly wage, but the correspondence course was a great incentive for a prospective student since "much time and expense can be saved by the student familiarizing himself with requisite technicalities before coming here."[45]

A University of Chicago comment, printed in the 1905 NICOO catalog, condoned correspondence courses by saying: "Experience has shown that such directions may be given a student by correspondence as will enable him to accomplish work of a high order."[46]

But they also added: "And while in no case should it be regarded as a substitute for class-room work, it may be well used to supplement it, at least by those who, for one reason or another, are prevented for a time from enjoying class-room privileges of instruction."[47]

By completing an additional 2-week classroom course, or a 6-week correspondence course, graduates could earn a Bachelor of Ophthalmology degree. Graduates of a third term, received a Master of Ophthalmology; and finally, after a fourth term followed by a thorough examination, a Doctor of Ophthalmology degree was awarded. All the course work was "exceedingly practical — just what the optician needs to do accurate fitting by the most improved methods and know what he is about all the time."[48]

Successful candidates received "an elegantly engraved diploma conferring the degree of Doctor of Optics. Those who are awarded advanced degrees receive special diplomas conferring such degrees. All diplomas are signed by the full faculty." Graduates also received an Alumni Association membership. With an impressive diploma and a state licensing board certificate mounted on the office wall, a practicing optometrist could assure his patients that he was truly a professional, and infinitely more qualified than a lens peddler or dispensing optician.[49]

The Alumni Association provided graduates with a supportive professional network. Reunions attracted alumni from all over the United States, Canada, and South America; and drew letters from graduates practicing in such remote places as New Zealand and Australia. More than mere social occasions, the 2-day reunions offered alumni an opportunity to attend lectures and seminars aimed at updating their skills and business practices.[50]

In 1908, NICOO was one of 42 independent optometry schools nationwide promising students a 6-month program guaranteed to prepare them to take the state licensing examinations.[51]

Two years later, New York City's Columbia University became the first American university to offer optometry courses. Their 2-year extension department program included a complete range of mathematical, scientific, and medical subjects which were taught by a number of eminent optometric educators including Drs. Andrew Jay Cross, Frederic A. Woll, and Charles F. Prentice.[52]

NICOO increased its tuition to $50 in 1914, but this didn't reduce enrollment: 30 students graduated that December. The school rented more floor space in the Masonic Temple Building in 1915, and added evening sessions to the schedule. Dr. James B. McFatrich died that year, and his brother George took on the burden of managing both successful family enterprises.[53]

DO IT NOW!

FROM THE MID-1880s to the 1900s the number of female physicians in the U.S. had increased from 2.6 to 5.6 percent: 7000 American women versus 258 British women were practicing medicine. NICOO had been training and graduating female students since the 1890s, and the alumni association regularly elected female officers throughout the 1900s.[54]

THE LARGEST AND
BEST EQUIPPED
IN THE WORLD

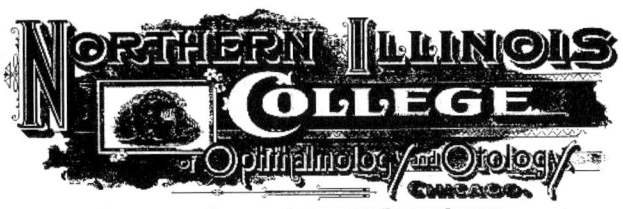

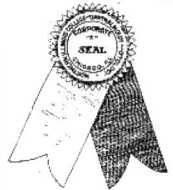

Elaborately-designed diplomas proudly displayed practitioners qualifications as Doctors of Optics, Bachelors of Optics, and Doctors of Ophthalmology. The Alumni Association certificate meant a practitioner was part of a professional brotherhood.

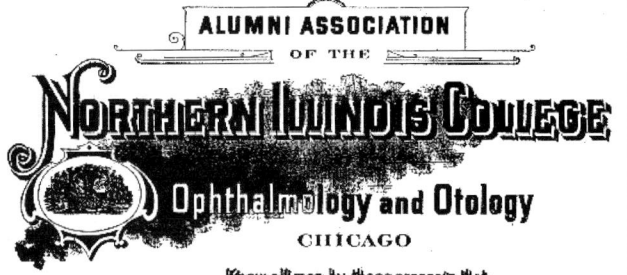

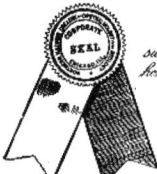

Dr. Ellen Colley, a 1913 NICOO graduate, was a typical example of the women who entered into private practice during the First World War. Colley was just one of a number of women who were not only AOA members, but held important positions as officers. State associations also welcomed female membership. Colley also became one of the Illinois Optometric Society's vice presidents. As early as 1904, the AOA's second vice-presidential post was held by a woman, and in 1907, so was the Physiological Section's vice presidential position.

As men entered the war in the spring of 1917, female enrollment at NICOO boomed. The school's correspondence courses were also a reasonable alternative for women seeking advanced education, and understandably the school took great pride in the quality of this program.[55]

Dr. George W. McFatrich described the flexibility which the school's curriculum offered prospective students in a September 28th 1917 letter to Mr. Wm. Greenberg:

> *We wish to call your attention again to our correspondence course which for its practical features is unsurpassed. One can thoroughly inform himself in optics by correspondence if he follows the directions laid down by the Northern Illinois College of Ophthalmology and Otology.*
>
> *Our course is complete and practical, which is thoroughly proven by the many graduates we have who are doing an extremely satisfactory business, having obtained their knowledge of optics through our correspondence and attendance courses. There is not one part of optics that we cannot thoroughly explain to you through our correspondence course. We do not send you written lectures but take the work up systematically by text books, the only true way to master any subject. You will find things you do not understand, these you will ask us about, and we in turn will thoroughly explain everything to you.*
>
> *Even if you expect to take an attendance course, the correspondence course is invaluable and costs you no more. It will save you time while in attendance, for having mastered your technical work, you can devote your time here to more practical work.*
>
> *Remember that our fee of $50.00 gives the matriculant the privilege of both attendance and correspondence courses. There is no pro-*

fessional calling which you can master so quickly, and it pays well. Why not begin at once? Remember the golden rule, "DO IT NOW".

Very truly yours,

G.W. McFatrich, M.D., President[56]

That same year, NICOO acquired the Chicago School of Refraction, increasing both the school's resources and student body.[57]

By year's end, Dr. George McFatrich resigned as the college's president and secretary. He split the positions between Dr. George A. Rogers (president) and Elva Maybee (secretary-treasurer), but still maintained a controlling interest in the school's stock. Rogers was an ideal choice. Besides being a longtime faculty member, Dr. Rogers was a regular contributor to *The Optical Journal and Review of Optometry*, a popular lecturer, author of a number of optometric books on subjects ranging from shadow tests to ophthalmic lenses, and a former president of the Illinois Optometric Society.[58]

As NICOO continued to grow, additional legislation and professional organizations spread across the nation. In 1924, the District of Columbia became the last continental territory to pass an optometric bill. The profession had firmly established itself in the United States.[59]

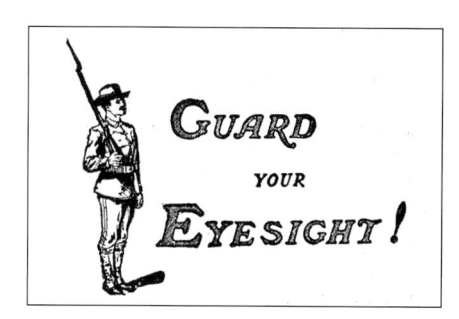

shadow test: a test which gives an approximate evaluation of the anterior chamber's depth. It is carried out by placing a penlight on the temporal side of the eye at the level of the pupil and directing the beam of light horizontally towards the inner side of the eye.

ophthalmic lens: a lens used to correct vision.

The profession began a series of public education campaigns geared to remind the public about the importance of vision care, a tradition that is still in practice today.

OPTOMETRY
IN AMERICA

38

Optical illusions have always been popular. But their usefulness is in vision treatment. SIRDS (single image random dot stereograms) are the latest technological advance. For an example, take a look at the end papers at the beginning and end of this book.

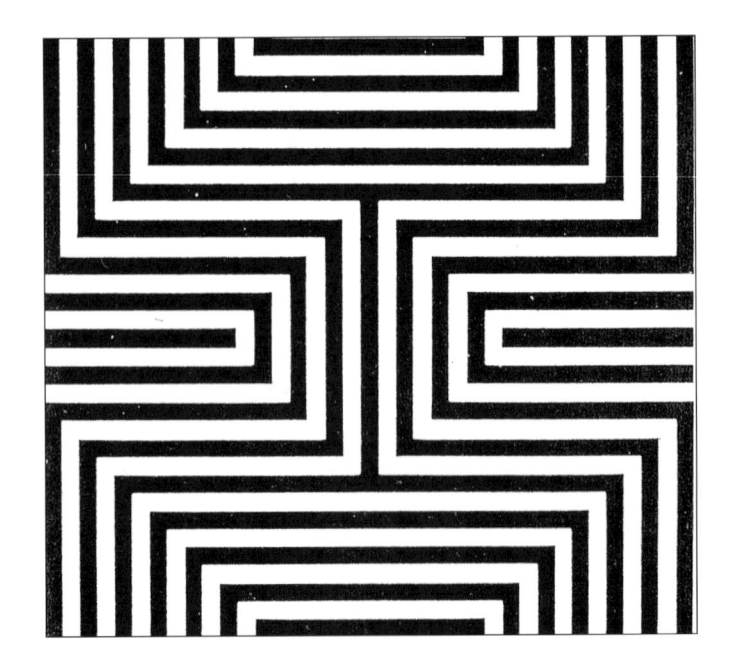

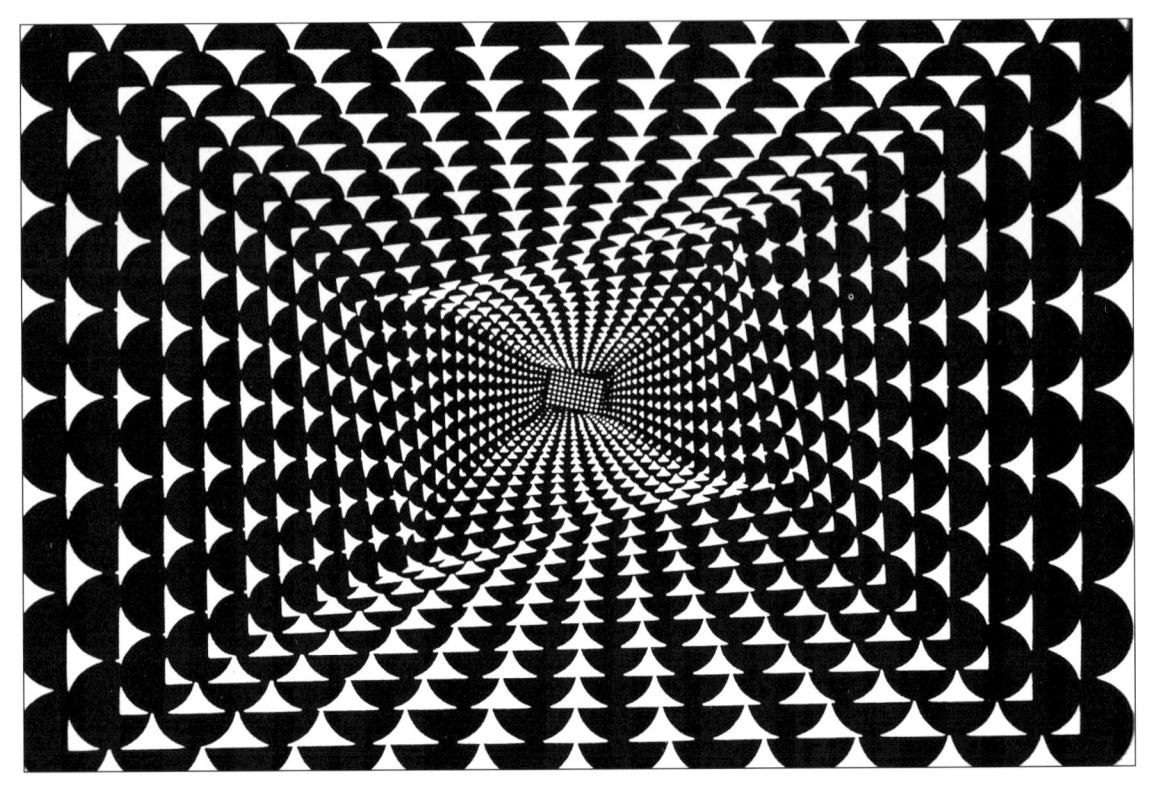

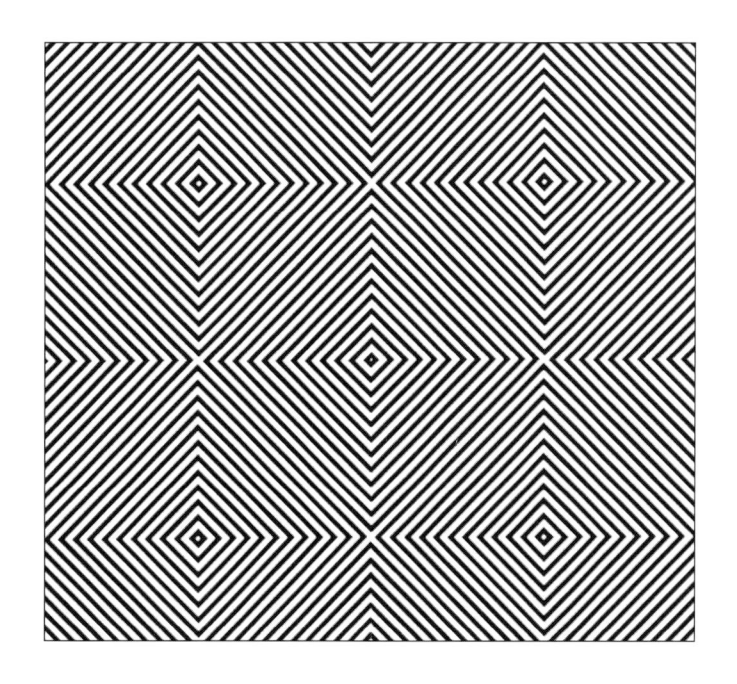

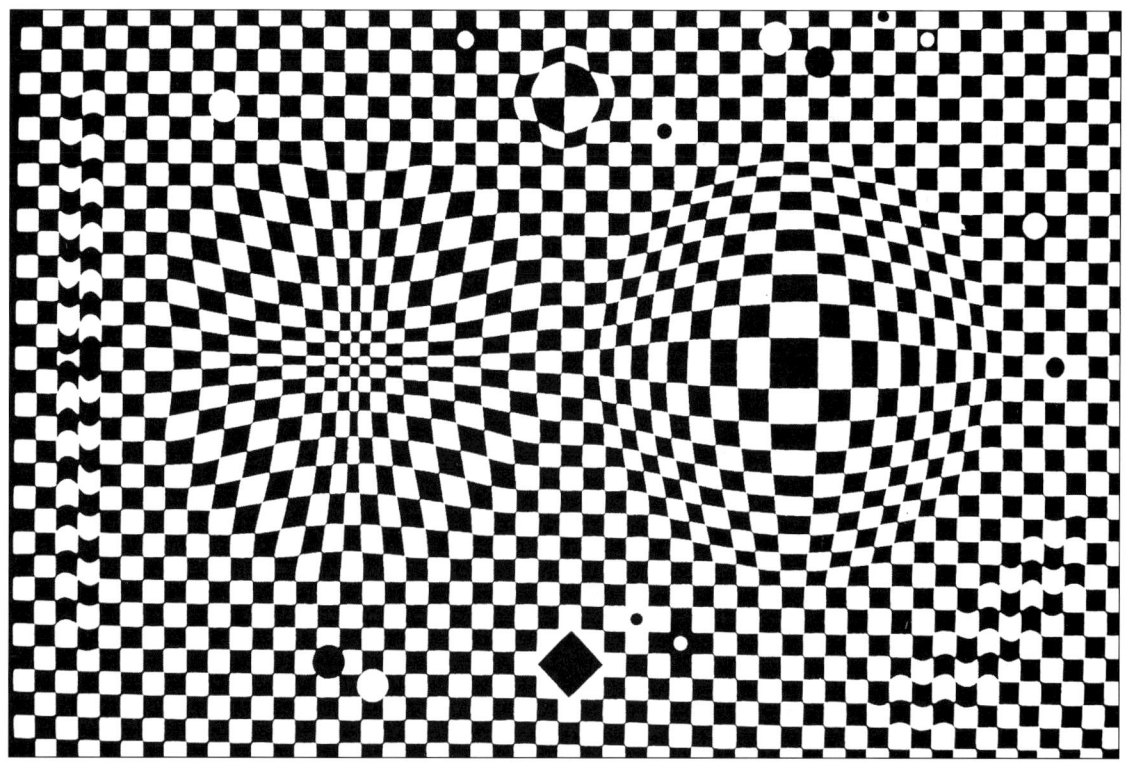

THE LARGEST AND
BEST EQUIPPED
IN THE WORLD

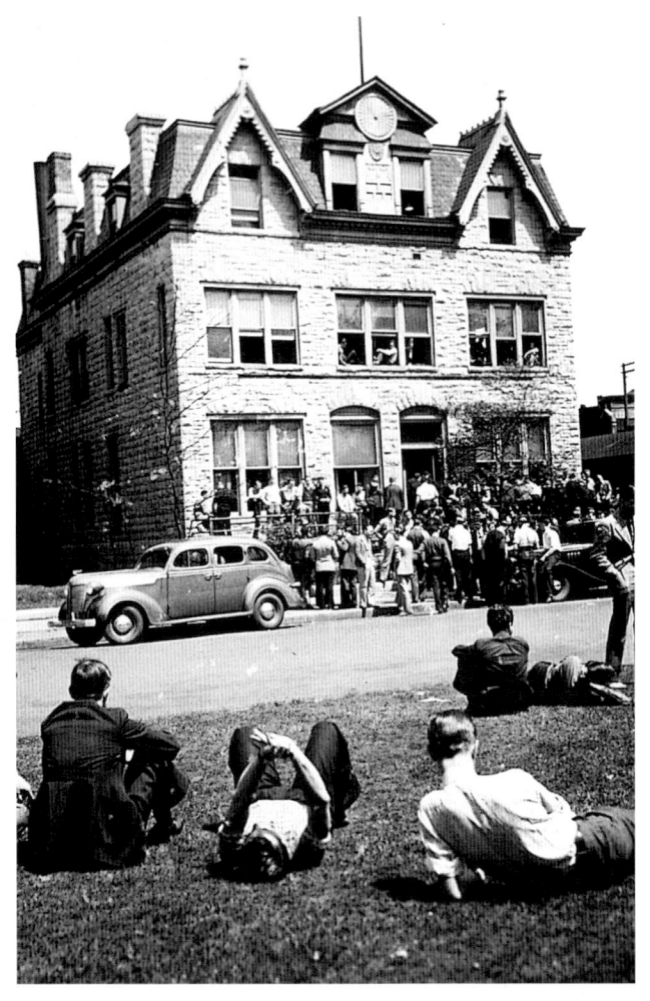

CHAPTER 3

Bring *on* Your State Boards!

NORTHERN ILLINOIS COLLEGE OF OPTOMETRY

THE ERA OF INSTRUMENTATION

AS A TEEN GROWING UP in Sedalia, Missouri, William Bray Needles worked in a small jewelry shop that sold spectacles. In 1899, he attended classes at Chicago's McCormick Optical College which had been founded 6 years earlier by Dr. Charles McCormick. The school offered both attendance and correspondence optical courses, and as one ad declared, the school could "teach more about eyes and nervous affection caused by them than any optical college."

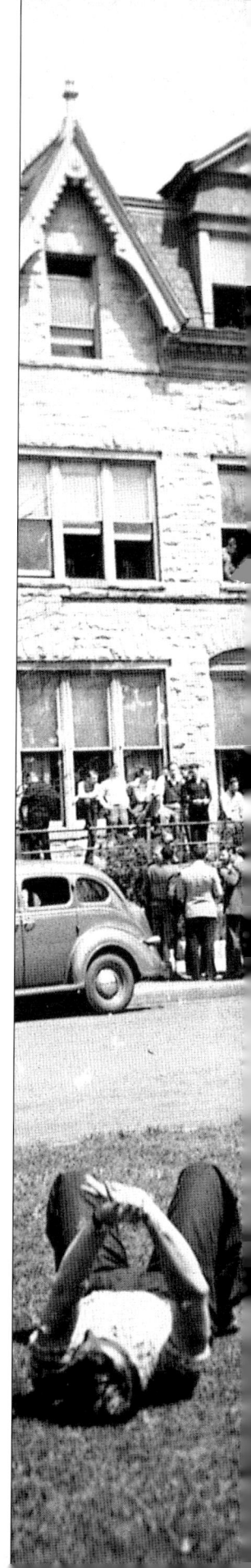

Northern Illinois College of Optometry's Drexel Boulevard campus offered students dormitory accommodations as well as "the largest physical plant dedicated to the teaching of optometry."

Dr. McCormick also published a book entitled *Optical Truths* which he used to promote both the profession and his school.[1]

After graduation, Dr. Needles opened optometric practice in Kansas City, Missouri. Troubled by his local colleagues' lack of professional knowledge Needles turned his attentions toward optometric education. He began to conduct a series of successful evening optometric lectures and workshops; accepted a teaching position at the Kansas City School of Optometry; and even taught refraction courses sponsored by the F.C. Merry Company. By helping to establish Dr. Needles as a teacher, the company hoped to ensure that more people would learn to use their trial cases.[2]

His classes were so successful that, in 1907, Needles founded his own school: the Needles Institute of Optometry. Three students enrolled in the first session, but the program and enrollment expanded rapidly, allowing Needles to incorporate his school in 1910.[3]

Five years later, the Needles Institute of Optometry had 7 faculty members teaching 30-week correspondence and attendance courses. In the early 1920s, the school offered a 2000-hour/2-year and a 1000-hour/1-year course in order to comply with the varying state laws. The school additionally conducted post-graduate and specialized courses for practicing optometrists.[4]

School texts like *Anatomy and Physiology of the Eye* (1919) and *Practical Work on the Extrinsic Muscles of the Eye* (1917) were written by Dr. Needles or the school's principal, Dr. Ernest Occhiena. These small, easily-comprehensible books were written for non-medically-oriented students.

As Needles and Occhiena wrote:[5]

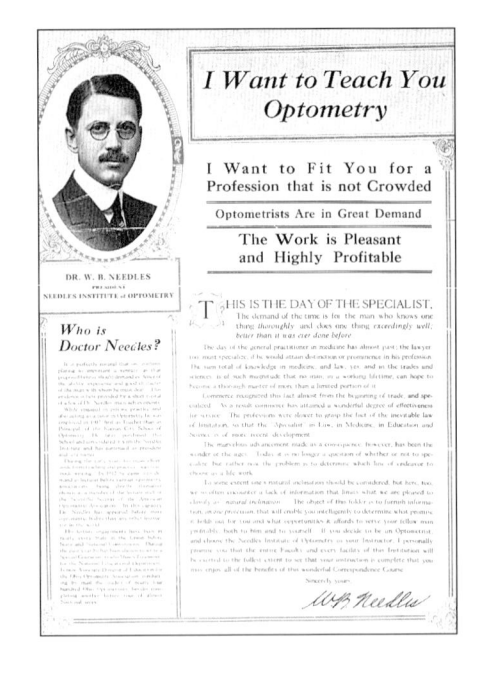

William B. Needles established his name with his Kansas City school and a busy nationwide lecture schedule.

Student testimonials were powerful recruitment tools.

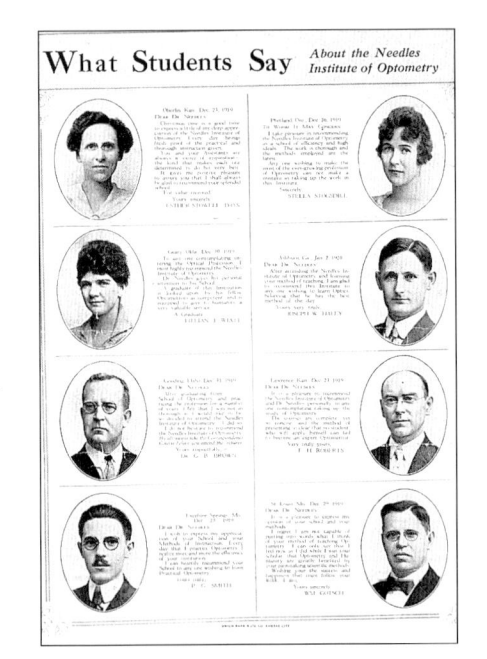

> *Optometrists and students who seek to improve their knowledge of the anatomy and physiology of the eye are sometimes embarrassed by the wealth of material available for study. Large volumes frequently baffle the seeker because of the difficulty of selecting essential information from them.*
>
> *This little textbook has been prepared after a plan approved by leading instructors in various sciences. The outline arrangement gives prominence to the more important features, thus focusing attention and making them easy to learn and retain.*[6]

This was reputedly optometry's "Era of Instrumentation," and the general adoption of objective testing procedures and improved examination equipment meant that practitioners no longer needed to rely on the patient's subjective responses to determine need. During the First World War, America became a leading manufacturer of optical products and equipment. (This was partly due to the disruption of European trade at that time.) Invisible bifocals and improved corrective lenses were additional innovations developed in that period. Consequently, students, practitioners, and the public had a lot more to learn about human vision and its care than could solely delivered in the classroom environment.[7]

With his school firmly established, Needles embarked on a highly-successful lecture circuit career as part of the AOA Department of Education's public education campaign. Orators specializing in just about any subject toured the country prior to the invention and popularization of radio and television. It was a popular form of entertainment — complete with booking agents, theater tours, and summer camps. Besides addressing local, state, regional, and national optometric conventions and community groups, Dr. Needles conducted optometric workshops nationwide, including a week-long seminar in 1916 at the University of California at Berkeley. He also tirelessly testified at state legislative hearings in favor of increased regulation of the optometric profession. And in his numerous articles on the subject, he repeatedly called for an increase in the number of qualified optometrists.[8]

Other state and private universities were also establishing optometric programs. Five years after Columbia University started their extension program, Ohio State Uni-

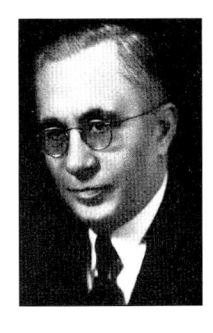

Dr. Ernest Occhiena worked with Needles at both the Kansas City and Chicago schools.

versity added a 4-year undergraduate course which conferred a Bachelor of Science degree in optometry. And in 1923, the University of California at Berkeley founded its own 4-year program.[9]

In a move similar to one made by the AMA's Council on Education in 1904, the International Association of Boards of Examiners in Optometry (later known as the International Board of Boards or IBB), in 1918, adopted a resolution that required all American optometry schools to only admit students who had completed 4 years of high school and received a diploma. The IBB also required optometric schools to adopt a minimum 1000-hour attendance course, which could be completed in 8 months (correspondence courses could no longer be offered). Lastly, the IBB strongly recommended that all independent optometry schools convert to non-profit status.[10]

During a 1921 Chicago speaking engagement Needles finally met Dr. George McFatrich, who offered him ownership of NICOO. McFatrich's interests in the Murine Eye Remedy Company made great demands on his time, and by then, Needles was one of the nation's most renowned optometrists and educators. After Dr. Needles agreed, Dr. McFatrich stated in an official announcement: "In Dr. W.B. Needles I recognized all of the elements of a successful educator, a man who will place the work of the college on even a higher plane than it has yet occupied."[11]

PIONEER OF THE LARGE SCHOOLS OF OPTOMETRY

DR. NEEDLES purchased NICOO's outstanding stock in 1922, and assumed the presidency. McFatrich stayed on as Professor of Ophthalmology and served as President Emeritus. In *The Optical Journal and Review of Optometry*, Dr. Needles proudly declared:[12]

> *It is with anticipation of much pleasure and no small degree of pride that I enter this new sphere of service. I have long appreciated the worth of the Northern Illinois College as the pioneer of the large schools of optometry and have known it to be an*

influential and well-conducted institution with a wide circle of friends. The great host of graduates of this college have had a large part in building the profession of optometry.[13]

Needles moved his family and practice to Chicago. He left the Needles Institute under the direction of Dr. Ernest Occhiena until the schools officially merged in 1926. That same year, Needles changed NICOO's name to Northern Illinois College of Optometry (NICO), and, in accordance with IBB recommendations, he re-chartered the school as a non-profit institution with himself as president/dean, and his sister, Lida, as secretary and registrar.[14]

Needles moved NICO from its trademark Masonic Temple Building to a former silent-movie studio on Drexel Boulevard located in Chicago's south side. The remodeled building included 9 lecture rooms, administrative offices, a clinic, a surgical amphitheater, and fully-equipped laboratories. In 1930, work was completed on a 5000-square-foot annex that housed a new clinic with 10 examination rooms and a 400-seat gymnasium/auditorium. The school advertised that its nearly 12,000-square-foot facility was "the world's most extensive plant for the exclusive teaching of optometry."[15]

NICO added a 2000-hour/2-year Doctor of Optometry degree to the curriculum, and the annual tuition was raised to $225. Both the Needles Institute of Optometry and NICO had been teaching the same philosophy of refraction, so the merged curriculum was not radically altered.[16]

Throughout the 1920s and 1930s, Dr. Needles publicly rallied against pressures he felt the state boards were imposing on optometric educators. He believed that if optometry was to survive as an independent profession — to compete against ophthalmologists and oculists — optometrists needed to join together to support and promote optometric education. In a 1925 *The Optical Journal and Review* article, Needles wrote:[17]

Dr. George McFatrich and the prominent physiologist Dr. W.D. Zoethout were among the early NICO faculty.

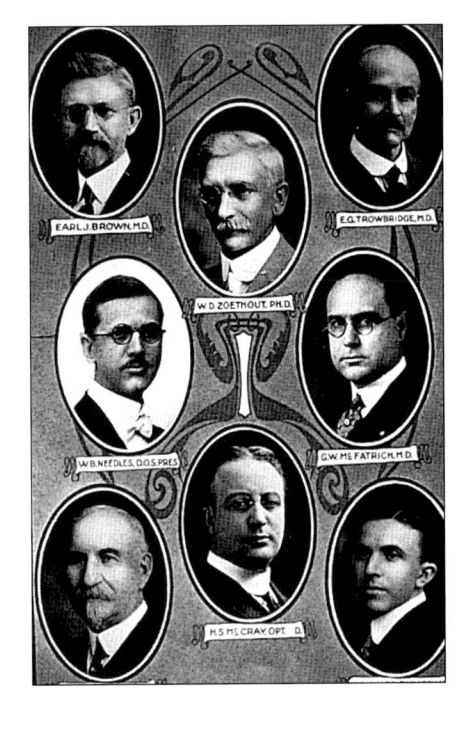

We need not care if medical men charge that our practitioners are too hastily trained. It does not matter what educators say. Our real concern is as to what the public thinks of us. Since they have patronized us and set up a profession, originally composed by "poor blind candidate," we need not fear but that they will support us increasingly and elevate us to the highest estate we can hope to reach, provided there are enough of us who are of the character being graduated by the optometry colleges of these days. We have not a school to spare. We need more, but at least we must encourage and support those we have, and put aside the "holier than thou" attitude which has been assumed by some men, themselves having the very flimsiest of educational backgrounds. The next few years will tell the story. We will go on to success, or fail, as we decide this great question."[18]

Needles contended with the IBB that "extraneous subjects" — English, history, and general sciences — were not necessary and were, in fact, harmful to the profession: they delayed students' entry into the field. He also feared that ophthalmologists would fill the vacuum created by an optometric shortage. But the AOA and IBB were more concerned with professional standing than the sheer output of qualified optometrists. Unlike other health professions, optometry had been associated with manufactured products in its infancy, not with service. Most medical and dental professions were far removed from product sales in the eye's of the public and the AOA, along with other affiliated associations, were determined to change that misconception of optometry as quickly as possible. [19]

Around that time the AOA reported that out of 18,467 registered American optometrists, 23.7 percent were AOA members. Motions were taken to refine the profession's scope — the AOA's Code of Ethics was enhanced to reflect the importance of doctor-patient relationships — and the IBB took a giant step: they started inspecting and rating the nation's optometry schools. By 1929, the IBB had accredited 7 schools including NICO which boasted nearly 15,000 alumni at that time.[20]

Eventually, Dr. Needles conceded to the IBB's demands. The 1933-1934 admission criteria complied with the latest IBB recommendations, and the degree program was increased to 3312 hours/3-years from the

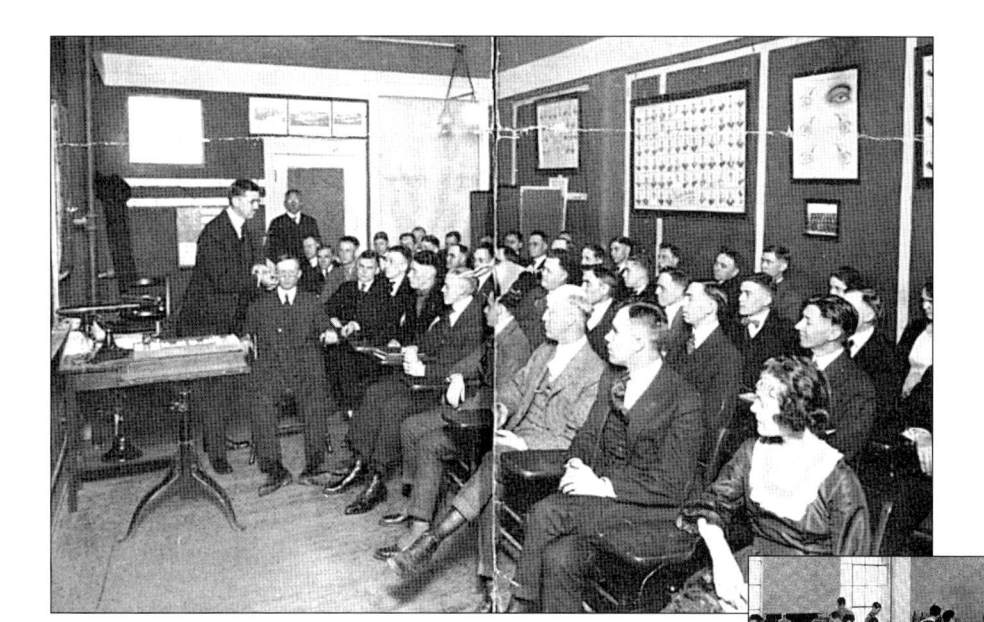

NICO students had the best available classroom and lab facilities.

earlier 2160 hour/2- year plan of the previous year.[21]

The IBB's demands were not entirely unfounded. During the 1920s, researchers discovered that human vision is not solely optically-based, but it is also a physiological function. Binocular vision, accommodation, convergence, and the phorias were being researched and analyzed in depth. Biological sciences — especially physiological optics — were becoming prominent in optometric education. Investigations conducted during the 1930s into optic nerves, cortical visual centers, and psychological optometry produced a wealth of additional information, further pressing the need for students to learn more than their predecessors.[22]

The new NICO curriculum covered an entire range of theoretical and practical optical and optometric courses as well as pathology, physiology, anatomy, psychology, economics, ethics, and clinical work. A semester-long course in optical mechanics also gave students a working knowledge of lens construction. Annual tuition increased to $300, with $40-115 for required equipment such as a retinoscope, ophthalmoscope, and a dissecting set. The key component of the new curriculum was clinical work: an internship program where students observed optometrists conducting patient examinations in the school's

binocular vision: a condition in which both eyes contribute to producing a single visual impression.

convergence: the turning of both eyes toward each other to focus on a single subject.

phoria: the direction of the focus line of one eye versus the other when there is no stimulus for both to fuse their images into a single impression.

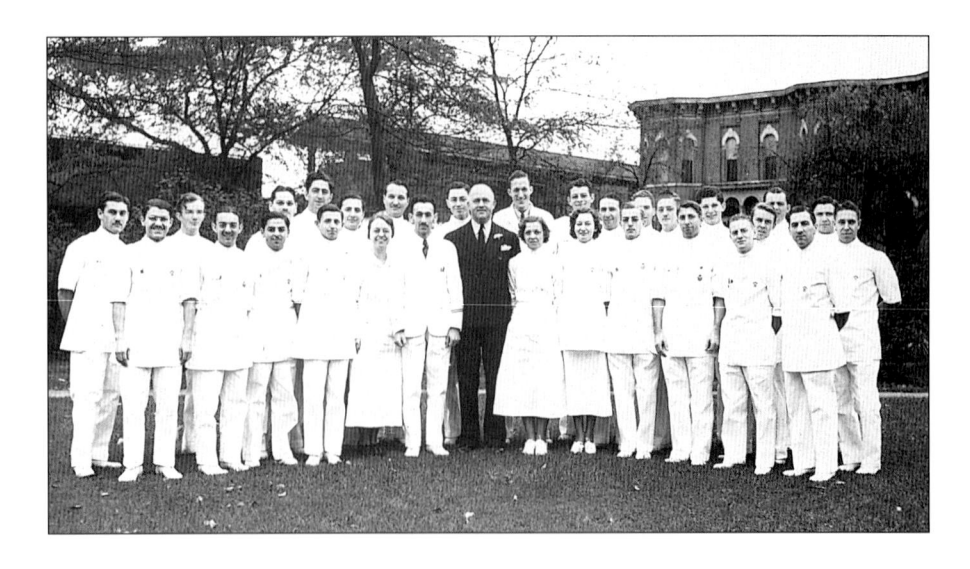

clinic and were later given hands-on, supervised training with real patients.[23]

As the 1930s catalog explained: "By means of this disciplined daily practice of scientific optometry sustained over a period of nine consecutive months, with a concurrent upbuilding of the sense of responsibility and a whetting of the appetite for continued research, it is the purpose of clinical courses…to turn out men and women who are eager for the exacting duties of their chosen calling, competent to cope with any eye case that may be presented to them, and imbued with that superb assurance which rests upon a smooth and facile technique backed by accurate and comprehensive scientific knowledge."[24]

Despite (or perhaps partially as a result of) the nation's economic downturn during the Great Depression, enrollment increased. Needles announced a 1934 expansion of NICO's faculty, curriculum, and physical plant. Plans for a new 3-story classroom/laboratory building were completed in 1937. The structure's ground floor, dedicated in 1938, housed a larger clinic with 25 general refraction rooms, a pathology amphitheater, plus diagnostic, dispensing and vision training rooms.[25]

As Needles' son, Dr. Richard Needles later recalled:

> *This was the first building ever constructed for the teaching of optometry. All others rented existing buildings. The state universities usually relegated the teaching of optometry to the basement of the physics lab or some other such distinguished location. This building was built*

Dr. Jerome Heather headed NICO's eye clinic, where students received hands-on training — conducting eye examinations with real patients.

entirely with private funds obtained from tuition (still $300 a year). There were no federal or state grants available nor was there an endowment fund of any type, nor aid from any alumni. Dr. Needles' name and monies he could borrow were the only resources.[26]

Needles also reorganized the school's departmental structure. He increased the faculty from 25 to nearly 50 professors, instructors, associates, and assistants, and created 4 separate divisions: Optometrical Sciences, Biological Sciences, Physical Sciences, and Social Sciences.

The Division of Optometrical Sciences — Theoretical, Technical, and Clinical Optometry Departments and the Northern Illinois Eye Clinic — was headed by Dr. Ernest Occhiena, who had also become NICO's dean.[27]

Dr. Carl F. Shepard, a Needles Institute of Optometry graduate who was self-taught in theoretical optometry, headed NICO's theoretical optometry department. Renowned for his research work in human vision, Shepard was also instrumental in the 1930 development of the Keystone stereoscope — a vision training device which was manufactured by the Keystone View Company, producer of home-entertainment stereoscopes and stereographs. (He also assisted in the development of many other vision training techniques during his career.)[28]

Shepard founded NICO's research department in 1923, and became the department's supervisor — a position he would hold for nearly 25 years. He also wrote numerous articles on the profession and was a regular contributor to *The Optometric Weekly*.[29]

The Optometric Extension Program, which provided "a means of building organization strength through educational features," originated in Oklahoma around 1930. This program of post-graduate clinics was orchestrated to help practitioners update their knowledge of the rapidly increasing body of theories and procedures.[30]

Dr. A. M. Skeffington, a 1915 Needles' Institute graduate, was a major architect of that program. Three years of divinity school training before he became interested in optometry more than adequately prepared him for his later role: he often substituted for Dr. Needles at professional and public speaking engagements. Skeffington gave radio talks and wrote numerous articles during the 1920s, promoting eye clinics for school children. From 1926 through

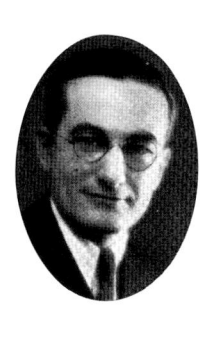

NICO faculty member Dr. Carl Shepard was best known for his work in vision training (orthoptics). He was also the developer of the Keystone

1928, Dr. Skeffington also established a series of post-graduate NICO summer courses.[31]

NICO's Biological Sciences Division — including the Physiology, Anatomy, Biology, Pathology and Bacteriology Departments — was headed by physiologist Dr. W.D. Zoethout. A Loyola University Medical School lecturer, Zoethout also authored *Physiology* (1931) which became a standard textbook, not only at NICO but at medical and dental schools nationwide.[32]

The school's Division of Physical Sciences, which encompassed both the Physics and Mathematics Departments, was headed by Dr. George B. Ruby; and the Division of Social Sciences, which included the Department of Psychology, was headed by Dr. Thomas G. Atkinson. The Ethics and Economics department was a separate section, which dealt with essential legal and business issues faced by practitioners.[33]

Besides working as an instructor in the Department of Ethics and Economics, Dr. W. Jerome Heather was NICO's Director of Clinics, whose faculty also included a recent NICO graduate, Dr. Irvin Borish (Chief of Staff); Dr. Thomas G. Atkinson (Pediatric Clinic); and Dr. Bernard

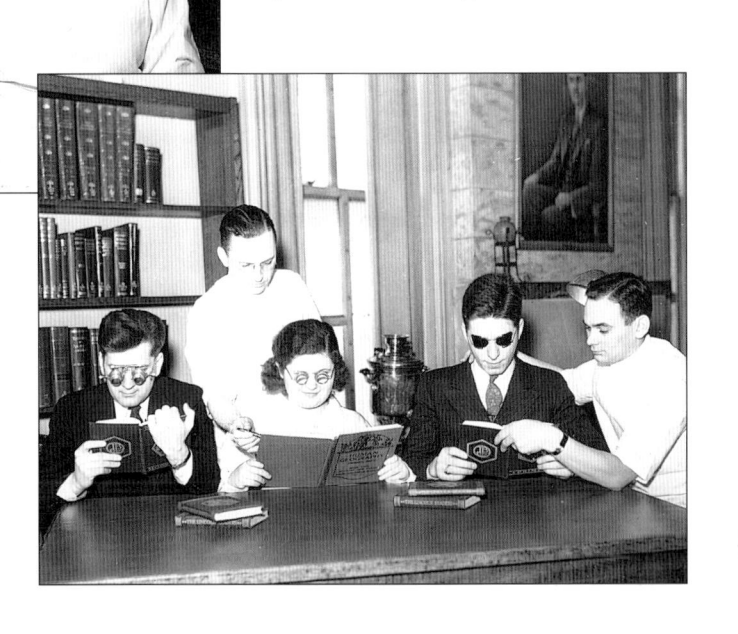

The Northern Illinois Eye Clinic offered both students and patients the best in state-of-the-art equipment and facilities for vision training.

Hoffmann (Ocular Pathology Clinic).³⁴

In the early 1900s, Manhattan ophthalmologist William H. Bates had developed a series of eye exercises which seemed to correct many of his patients' problems without surgery or corrective eyewear. Bates' theories were generally regarded by the medical community as radical diatribes bordering on heresy, and he was dropped from AMA membership in 1912. The Bates Method was the product of extensive eye muscle and vision training (orthoptics) research. Bates published both his theories and practical exercise procedures in a book entitled *The Cure of Imperfect Sight by Treatment Without Glasses* (1920). Orthoptics rapidly gained public approval after that. One of Bates' most ardent admirers was the famed British author and critic Aldous Huxley who had been diagnosed with partial blindness caused by keratitis while studying at Eton. Despite his limited vision, Huxley managed to graduate from Oxford, but was determined to find a cure for his problem. Huxley learned the Bates method from a friend, Margaret Corbett, and his sight gradually improved. He documented his positive experiences in two works: *The Perennial Philosophy* and *The Art of Seeing*. Another of Huxley's friends, Olive Brown, established a successful orthoptics practice based on Bates' vision training methods.³⁵

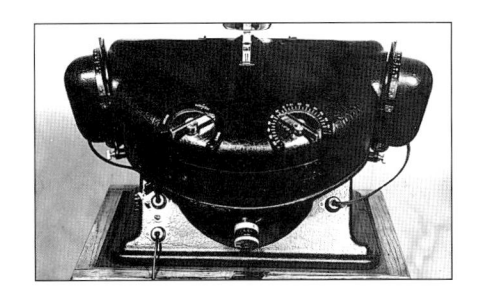

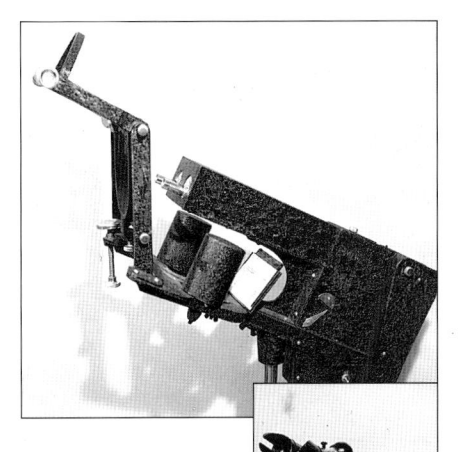

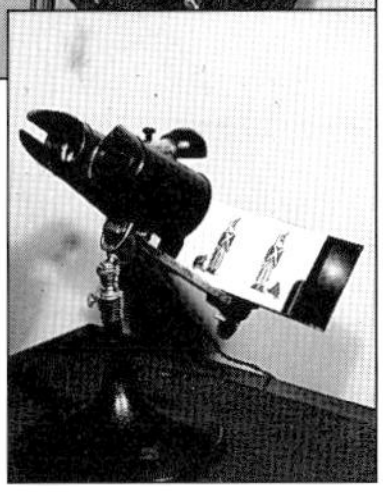

During the 1920s, interest in orthoptics also grew within the American optometric community. "The profession was growing more conscious of its services and 'playing down' the spectacle-selling aspect it had always attached to it."³⁶ Orthoptics was found to be a particularly viable treatment for strabismus, amblyopia, and squinting. The Northern Illinois Eye Clinic leapt ahead of its competition, by providing training for stu-

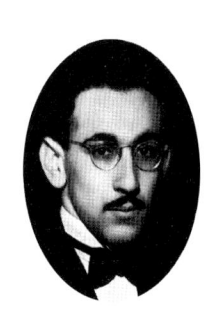

Strabismometers and telebinoculars were developed for use in orthoptics on patients with strabismus and astigmatism.

BRING ON YOUR STATE BOARDS!

Shortly after his graduation from NICO, Dr. Irvin Borish was hired as Clinic Chief of Staff.

RIGHT: Under the direction of Dr. Heather and the rest of the clinic's faculty, students were taught how to detect numerous pathologies.

BELOW: The clinic's professional examining rooms contained the latest in measuring equipment.

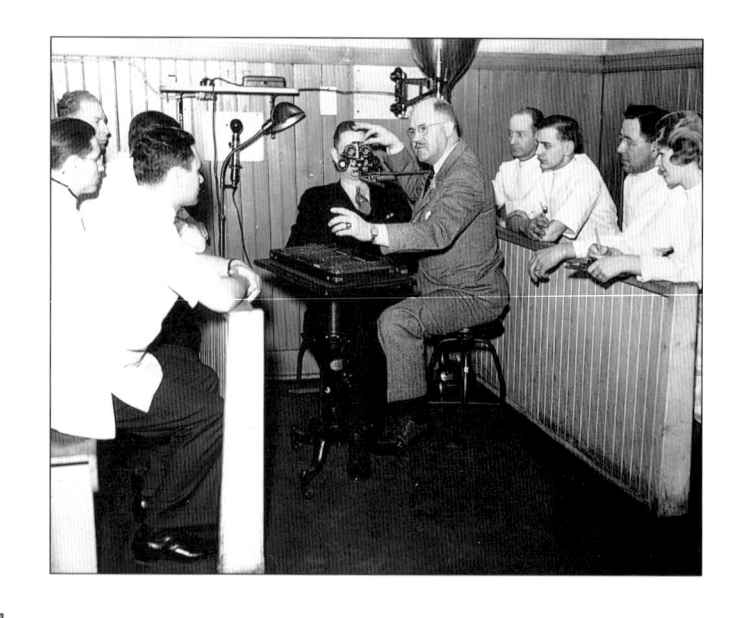

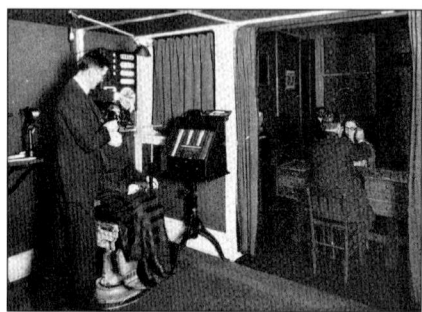

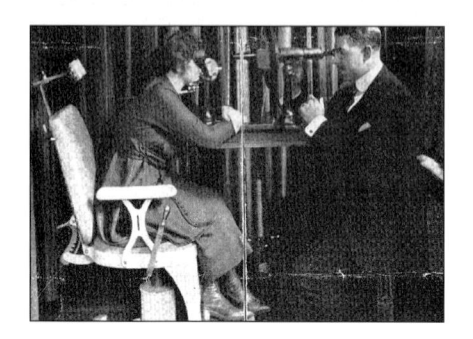

dents and treatment for patients with the latest orthoptic techniques and equipment.[37]

With the onset of the Great Depression, the clinic became one of the world's largest vision correction facilities, incorporating state-of-the-art diagnostic and treatment methods like orthoptics. Nearly 150 students and faculty began working with patients from the surrounding schools and welfare agencies in 1932. The list of relief organizations was extensive, and grew in 5 years to include: the Cook County Bureau of Public Welfare, Family Relief Association, Goodwill Agency, Hull House, Illinois Emergency Relief, Juvenile Court, Sacred Heart Church, Salvation Army, United Charities, Veterans' Bureau, and Women's Municipal Home.[38]

The clinic introduced optometric services to thousands of residents whose eyes had never been examined before, improving the public's vision while also providing critical student training: they spent more than twice as many hours working in the clinic than other students nationwide. And the clinic's community service was so valuable that during the Second World War the school's clinicians were deferred from military service.[39]

strabismus: a term for a cross-eyed condition in which both eyes don't focus on the same object at the same time.

amblyopia: a term for low vision acuity (20/30 or less) not due to poor focus, disease, or faulty eye structure.

squinting: a condition where the eye muscles attempt to force focus by narrowing or compressing the range of vision.

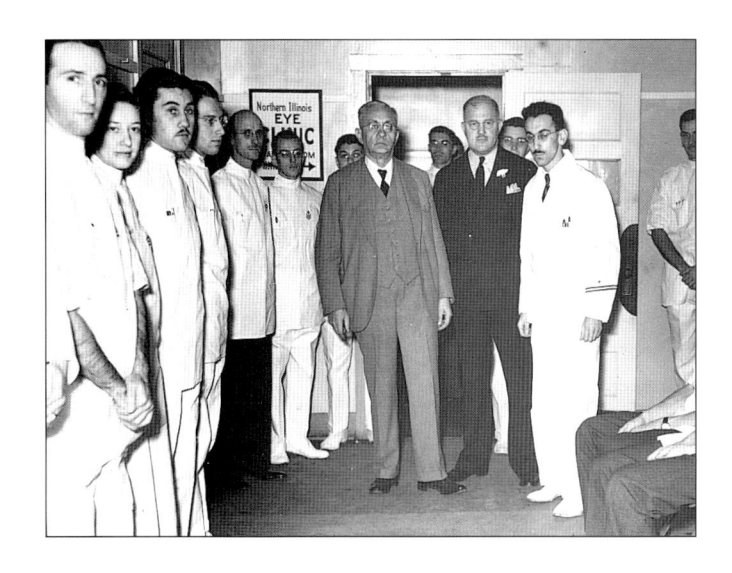

ABOVE: Drs. Occhiena (center) and Heather (right) regularly made rounds at the Northern Illinois Eye Clinic.

RIGHT: Many of the Depression-era patients to the clinic were referred by area social agencies.

Basic examinations included taking a full patient history, objective monocular and binocular testing, and diagnosis which cost patients 25 cents. (Although in most cases, the fee was reimbursed by a referring agency.) Additional dispensing and vision training programs were also carried out at the facility. In this comprehensive setting, students gained practical experience, not only in refraction and vision training techniques, but in patient-practitioner relations and in the detection of a wide range of ocular pathologies.[40]

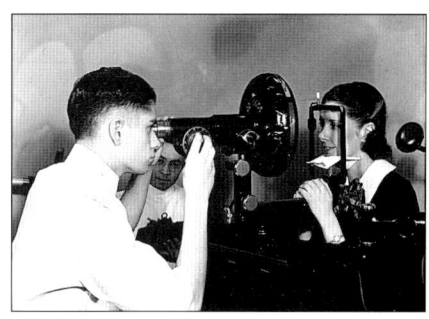

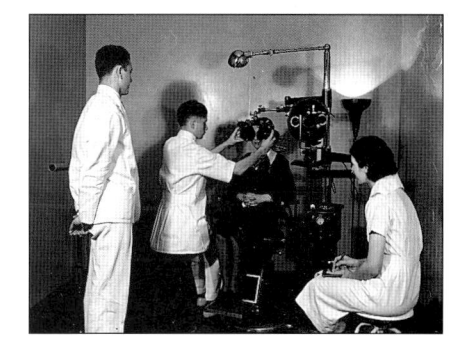

monocular tests: diagnostic testing of each eye's individual ability to focus.

binocular tests: diagnostic testing of both eyes' ability to focus together.

DIARY OF A MODERN INTERNE

WHILE EDUCATION was improving, so was life outside the classroom for optometry students. By 1931, NICO had 4 optometric fraternities — Omega Delta, Phi Theta Upsilon, Omega Epsilon Phi, and Mu Sigma Pi — which sponsored programs like lectures by professionals in the field, as well as standard academic social activities. Other extra-curricular groups included a masonic organization (the Square and Compass

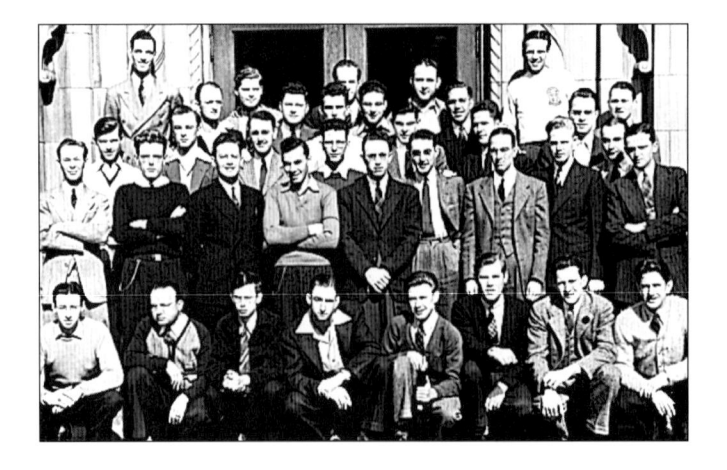

The Omega Delta fraternity (above) was just one of the optometric fraternities chartered on the NICO campus.

Club) which promoted "good fellowship among its members and with non-member students;" a Catholic fraternal organization (The Columbus Club); and a senior class honor society (the Tomb and Key).[41]

Golf, bowling, and tennis clubs as well as a varsity basketball team made up the sports program. The basketball team —their jersey was emblazoned with a large, anatomically complete eye — even had a few championship years before it was disbanded in favor of other activities.[42]

Many students lived in neighboring hotels like the Bernhard Hotel and the Hyde Park YMCA — which offered both room and board — until 1936, when the school acquired the Bernhard Hotel and opened its first dormitory. From that point on, all non-resident students moved onto the NICO campus. (Room and board costs at the time were $7.50-10 per week.)[443]

The 1937-1938 NICO catalog proudly listed a 659-person student body — 34 of whom were female. Among the 46 graduates in 1936, 7 women were listed including one magna cum laude graduate. Throughout the 1930s, NICO continued encouraging female applicants to join the profession in their catalogs. (NICO's support of women was also evident when the Alpha Chapter of Phi Kappa Rho, a national optometric sorority, was founded at at the school in 1928.)[44]

An article entitled "The Diary of a Modern Interne" appeared in *The Focus* 1933 yearbook. Authored by an anonymous student, this essay summarized the 1930s NICO experience:

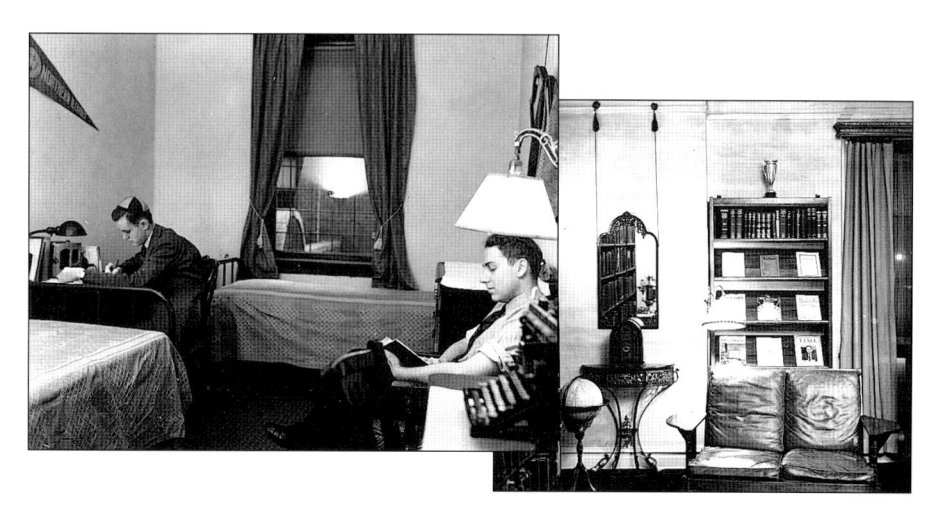

NICO's dormitory was originally the Bernhard Hotel. Room and board, plus facilities like the student lounge allowed students to concentrate on their studies without the worry of locating an apartment.

I have been looking forward for over two years to the time when my actual school work would be completed, and now that it has arrived I have a vacant sort of feeling. Leaving the friends I have made and good old NIC[O] wasn't considered when I was wishing for graduation day to come around. Neither was the idea that when school is finished the real work just starts. My clinical records show over three hundred hours of actual refraction and nearly three hundred patients in that length of time. I wonder how many newly graduated men can equal this.

There are some things that leaving Chicago cannot deprive me of, though, and they are knowledge of optometry, clinical experience second to none, and the old confidence to go out and build an ethical and successful practice regardless of the existing conditions.

Bring on Your State Boards!"[45]

National unemployment figures rose, in 1933, to 12.8 million Americans, representing roughly 25 percent of the work force. A 1929 California State Board of Optometry survey reported that the average optometrist earned $7500 a year, but 3 years later, like other health care professionals, few practicing optometrists were making that amount. And though there was as much demand for optometrists as ever, income prospects for new graduates grew slim.[46]

NICO didn't reflect these hard times. In 1933, there was a larger graduating class than ever before: 178 students. Student enrollment averaged about 400 people from 1927 to 1937; and by 1938, the student body nearly doubled to 700 enrollees. As Dr. Irvin Borish recalled, "What happened in the Depression was surprising; all colleges did very well. I guess, when you have high unemployment, you send everybody to college."[47]

The AMA Council on Education warned medical schools against admitting too many students during those years. They also encouraged state medical licensing boards to adopt tougher regulations on immigrating foreign physicians. Both of these actions served to reduce the ranks of the medical community while optometry's numbers grew.[48]

In keeping with additional IBB recommendations, NICO enhanced its curriculum by adding a fourth year, in 1938, which concentrated almost entirely on clinical work. To meet the public demand for more optometrists and Dr. Needles' own dictates, NICO switched from semesters to a quarterly system. Introduced by Dr. Irvin Borish, the transition facilitated students who wanted to finish their coursework in 3 years. Not all schools were able to make such a radical transition. By the late 1930s, NICO was one of only 8 remaining fully-accredited optometry schools in the nation.[49]

In 1941, the AOA implemented strict new educational guidelines, adopting the *Manual of Accrediting Schools and Colleges of Optometry* written by NICO faculty members Dr. Irvin Borish and Dr. Eugene Freeman. The AOA Council on Education and Professional Guidance was now responsible for accreditation. This same year, and under these new stricter guidelines, NICO received full accreditation.[50]

But a new and greater uncertainty suddenly faced the nation with the advent of the Second World War. "I'll never forget. We were in the offices of William Needles, president of Northern Illinois College of Optometry ... when President Roosevelt delivered his famous 'Day in Infamy' speech. We all sat down and listened to the radio wondering where the next few years would take us," AOA Secretary Ernest Kieknapp recalled. The AOA's Board of Trustees had convened in Chicago to plan the profession's future. Enrollment steadily declined between 1942 and 1943. (Most prospective and current students joined the war effort.) By 1944, there were only 60 students. Tragically,

Dr. Needles was stricken, in 1942, with heart disease. The 63-year-old doctor retired to play golf until his death. Dr. Occhiena also retired that year from his post as dean.[51]

In April of the same year, the U.S. Congress passed the G.I. Bill of Rights guaranteeing veterans educational funding on their return along with other financial aid. When the veterans came home in 1945, NICO and other educational institutions nationwide received a much needed boost. Enrollment soared to 2100 students by 1947.[52]

THE START OF A NEW LIFE AND THE END OF AN EMPIRE

THERE WERE SOME incoming students during the 1940s who did not have the advantages of the G.I. bill nor family to help see them through their education. These were incoming refugees — civilians escaping the torment of the battlefront and concentration camps in Europe and Asia, seeking new lives and careers in the United States. One example was a 1944 NICO graduate, Dr. Frederick Kushner. Born in Austria to Hungarian and Polish parents, he had studied medicine at the University of Vienna before the Nazi occupation. Kushner had been expelled from school as a result of anti-Semitic sentiments. He was even placed in a concentration camp, but he was fortunate and escaped to Great Britain the day before war broke out in 1939.[53]

Thanks to a family friend he managed to gain documents and passage to the United States, in 1940, where his mother and sister had already emigrated. Kushner spoke very little English at that time, so he accepted whatever work he could find after landing at Ellis Island. He found a job in the Mobile, Alabama shipyards. As previously mentioned, medical and dental schools and state examining boards were barring immigrants from entering school or practicing medicine in the United States during those years. Kushner wanted to continue his medical education but neither medical nor dental schools would even interview him.[54]

He got married in New Orleans, where he managed to find another job in the shipyards. When he began developing headaches on the job, his co-workers suggested he see an optometrist. There weren't any optometrists in Europe, and Kushner had no idea what optometry was. But he went as recommended for an examination at a department store that had an optometrist on premises. As Kushner remembered in an interview: "While he was examining me, I saw that he had gold cufflinks and that he had a gold pin on his tie. I looked around and could see that there was money there. I looked at him and said, 'Give me a job. I'd like to work here.' But he said, 'You have to go to school.'" The optometrist, a NICO graduate, sent Kushner to the library to get the names of American optometric schools. He wrote to all of them, but only Northern Illinois College of Optometry responded.[55]

Unfortunately, NICO could not accept him because he did not have a high school diploma. The European educational system did not have high schools per se, though the education level was generally better than that in the United States. He had his medical college academic records from the University of Vienna, but he did not have a high school diploma. But Kushner was still determined. He visited a Chicago Catholic school where the mother superior, after listening to his plight, decided to personally teach him English and other subjects necessary to get a high school diploma. He earned his diploma, and was finally accepted because of it by NICO dean, Dr. C. Stanley McGuire. After graduation, Dr. Kushner remained at the school, first becoming an instructor in the anatomy laboratory; later becoming assistant dean, interim dean and finally, in 1950, he became dean of the school.[56]

The biggest problem NICO administrators faced after the Second World War was the college's rapid growth. Once able to house the entire college, NICO's building was now needed solely to house the administration and was part of a six-building campus. "Old Main" contained the library, cafeteria, the student lounge, and ground-floor clinic space besides providing student housing. In August 1947, the school purchased the nearby First Church of Christ Scientist building, an impressive 2-story Greek Revival stone structure with a 1200-seat auditorium capped by a tall dome, where the school held assemblies, lectures, and graduation ceremonies.[57]

BRING ON YOUR
STATE BOARDS!

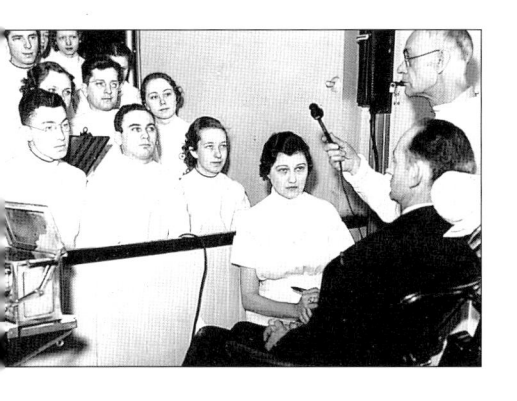

59

To accommodate the large influx of students after the war, NICO enlarged their facilities including an amphitheater, labs, and clinic space.

The upper stories of a former masonic hall with a street-level mortuary became Boydston Hall, housing the research department, classrooms, and labs. Greenwood Hall and the upper stories of the Oakland Building were also adopted for school use.[58]

To keep the growth orderly, NICO commissioned Dr. Howard Egan of Loyola University, Dr. Francis Shonka from the University of Chicago, and Dr. C.D. Turner of Northwestern University to survey its program and facilities. Dr. Egan, who led the survey team, proposed a new program that so impressed both the AOA and NICO's administrators that, in 1947, he was made dean of the school. Dr. Carl Shepard, who had returned to the school after his brief tenure as the dean of a competing school, headed a revival of the school's research department.[59]

During the late 1930s and throughout the Second World War, the Northern Illinois Eye Clinic served a total of 41,260 patients. By 1948, 26,000 patients were being treated in one year alone. That same year clinic fees were cut from $2 to $1, while lab work and eyewear were dispensed at cost to increase patient volume, giving students as many opportunities as possible to work directly with patients.[60]

The clinical staff — 22 optometrists, and 12 administrative assistants — were directed by Dr. Needles' nephew, Dr. James Grout, who had been appointed to the position in 1943. In 1948, Dr. Grout appointed Dr. Edward Friedlander as Chief of Clinic Staff.[61]

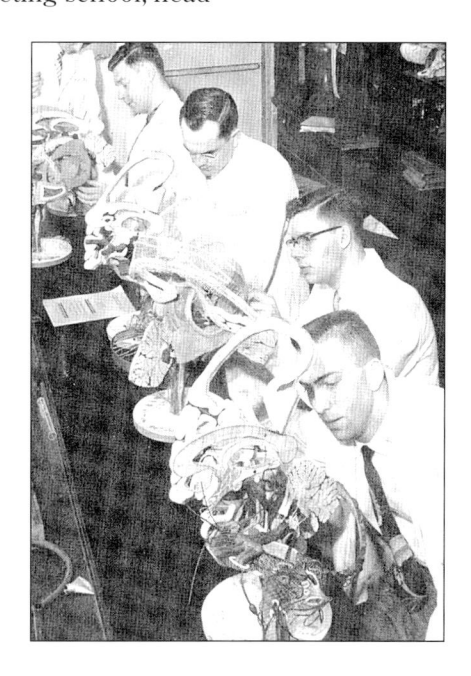

The September 1950 commencement exercises celebrated the graduation of 257 students, but the school also mourned the loss of one of its leaders as Dr. William B. Needles died that year. After a year of administrative transitions, Needles' son, Dr. Richard Needles, was appointed president (a position he held until November, 1951).[62]

In 1950, Dr. Richard Feinberg, a University of Rochester optometric program graduate and former dean of Pacific University's College of Optometry, came to NICO, replacing Dr. Richard Needles as the school's president: the first NICO president who was not a Needles family member.[63]

Another historic event took place in the late 1940s. The AMA lifted their 14-year ban prohibiting ophthalmologists from lecturing at optometric institutions. It was a sign that the relationship between the health care professions could eventually improve. As a result, NICO installed 10 additional examination rooms, specially equipped for a new staff of consulting ophthalmologists. But the winds of change were not stilled as the nation and the world entered a new decade of relative peace.[64]

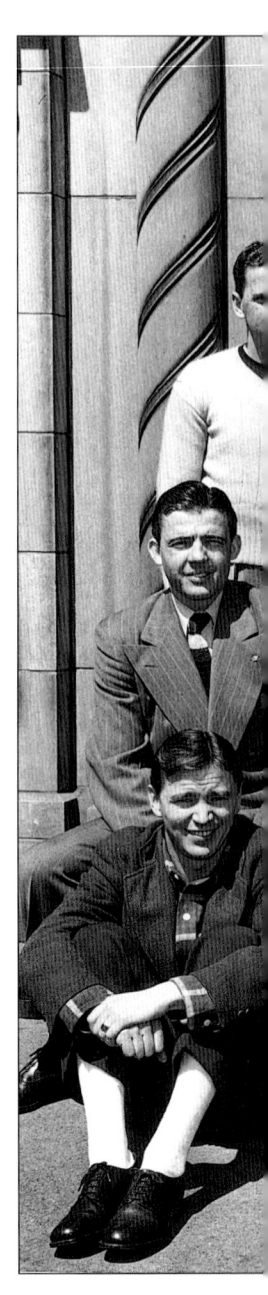

FACING PAGE:
Dr. Carl Shepard (second row, center) returned to NICO to head research department, pictured here with some of his students.

BRING ON YOUR
STATE BOARDS!

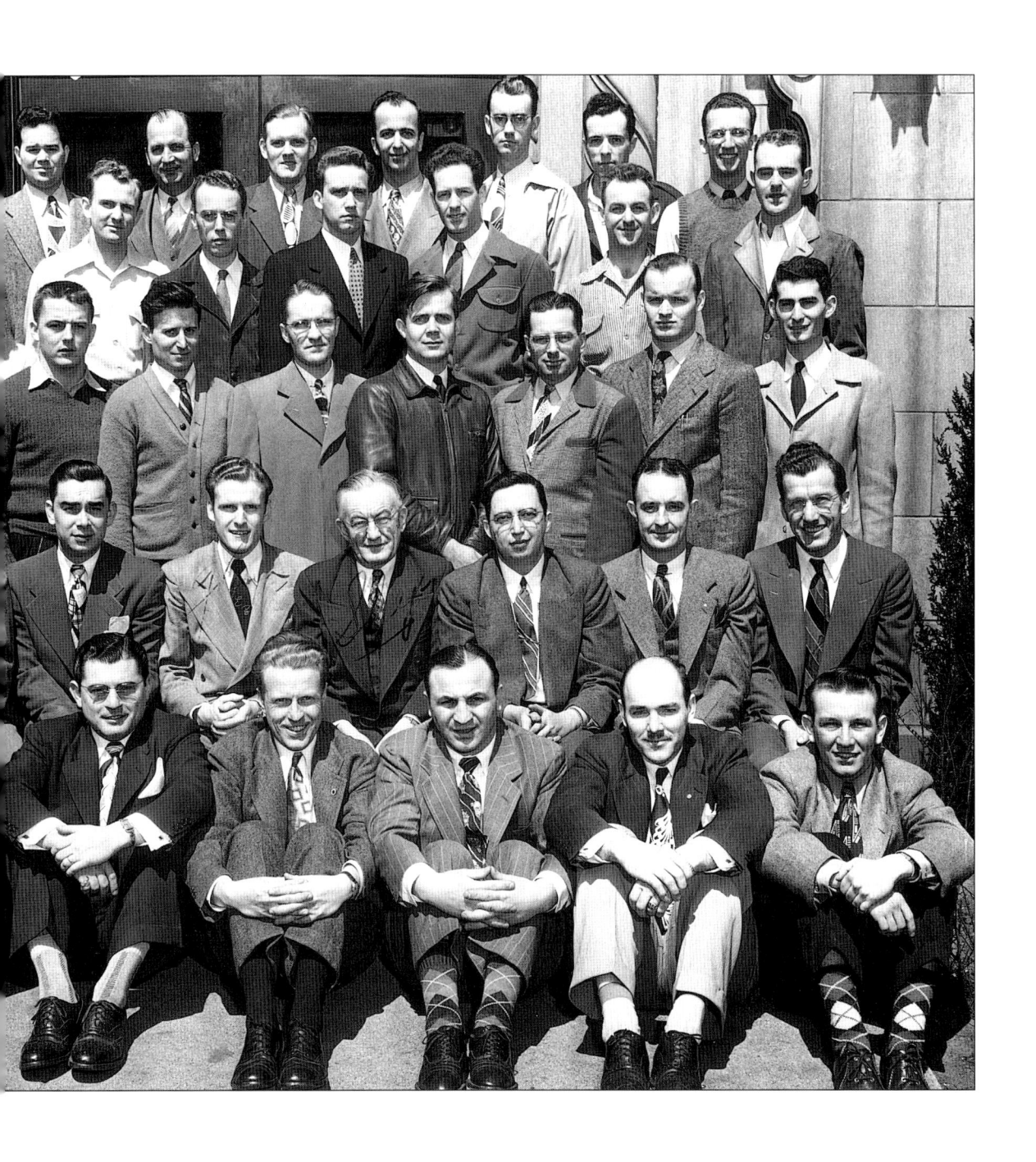

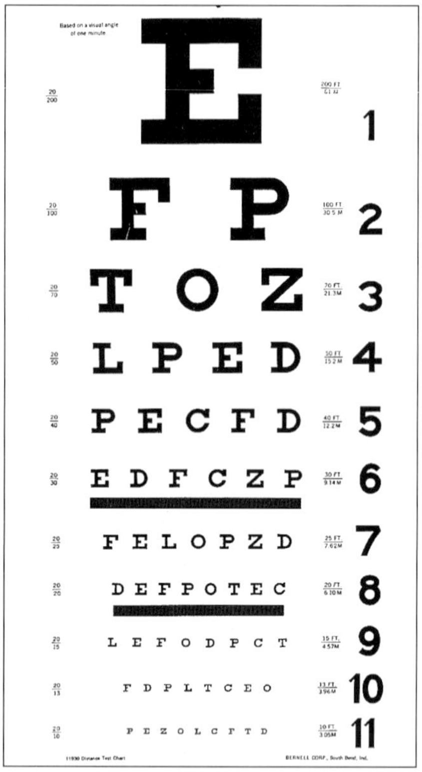
E
1
F P
2
T O Z
3
L P E D
4
P E C F D
5
E D F C Z P
6
F E L O P Z D
7
D E F P O T E C
8
L E F O D P C T
9
F D P L T C E O
10
P E Z O L C F T D
11

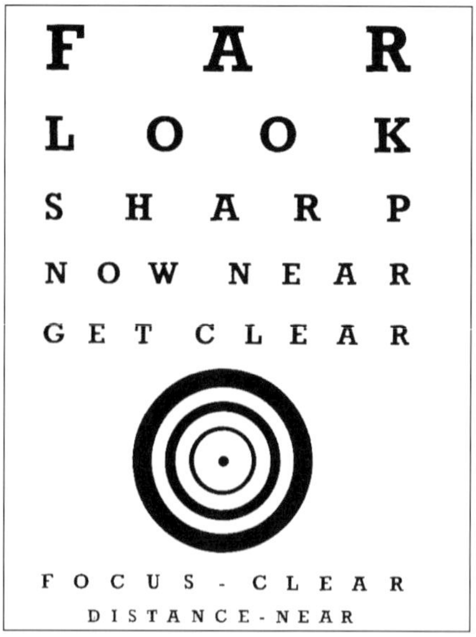
F A R
L O O K
S H A R P
N O W N E A R
G E T C L E A R
F O C U S - C L E A R
D I S T A N C E - N E A R

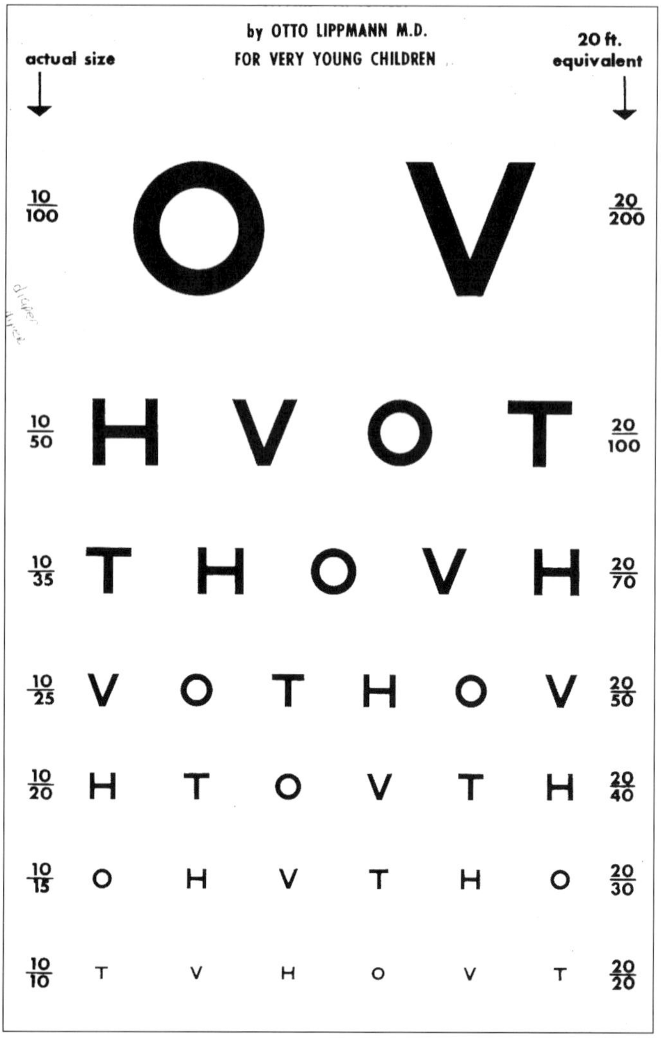
by OTTO LIPPMANN M.D.
FOR VERY YOUNG CHILDREN
actual size
20 ft. equivalent
10/100 O V 20/200
10/50 H V O T 20/100
10/35 T H O V H 20/70
10/25 V O T H O V 20/50
10/20 H T O V T H 20/40
10/15 O H V T H O 20/30
10/10 T V H O V T 20/20

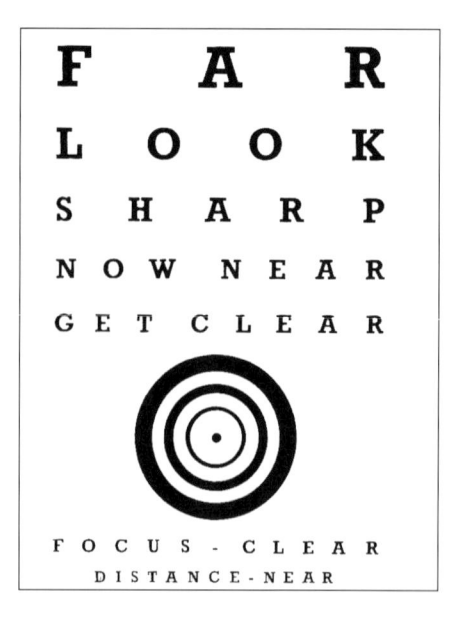

BRING ON YOUR
STATE BOARDS!

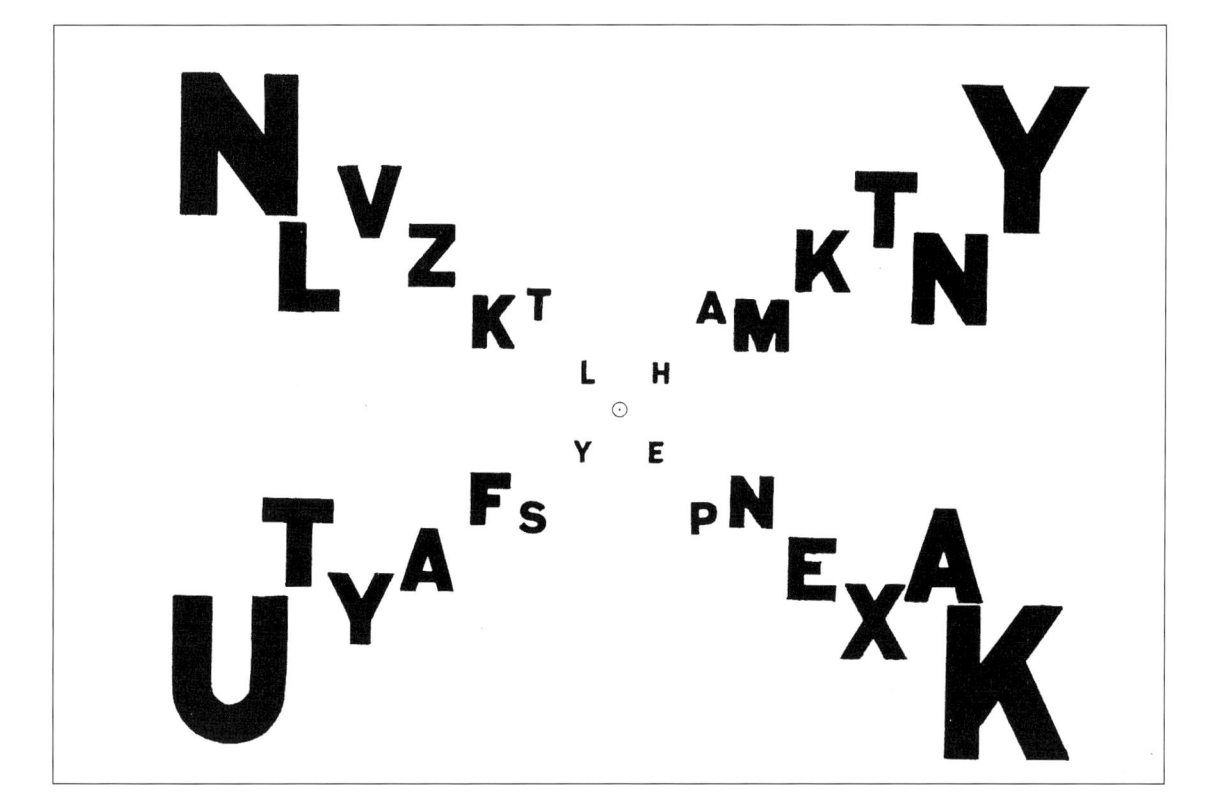

A variety of eye charts, based on Herman Snellen's 1863 designs (far left), were specifically designed to detect angular, shape, and size flaws in vision. The term 20/20 vision is derived from Snellen's observation that at a distance of 20 feet, a patient can read a certain line on the chart without visual aids. Snellen's charts are still in use today.

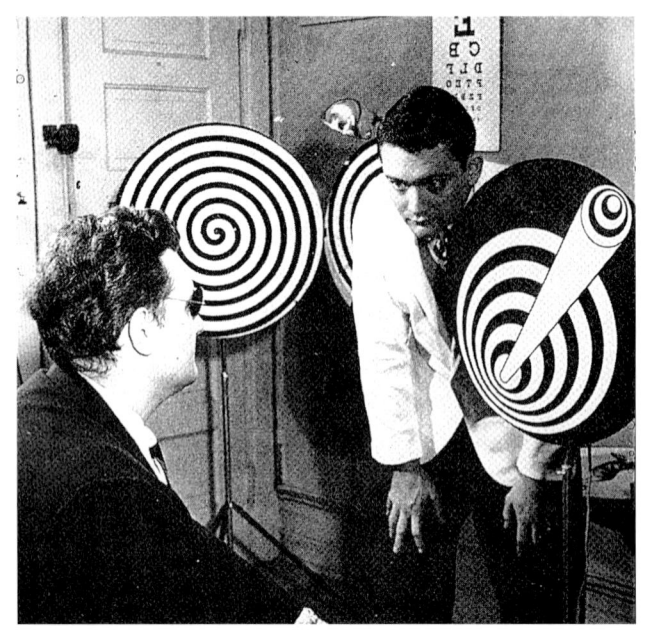

CHAPTER 4

EYES RIGHT

CHICAGO COLLEGE OF OPTOMETRY

A SIRLOIN STEAK WITH A FEW POTATOES

Vision training had become an important part of optometric treatment.

CHICAGO WAS HOME of the nation's largest school of optometry by the 1920s, but during the next decade, a competing institution emerged on the city's north side. In 1926, the same year that Dr. William B. Needles established the Northern Illinois College of Optometry, Reuben Seid graduated from the University of Illinois with a degree in medicine. After completing his internship at Michael Reese Hospital, Seid attempted to establish a medical practice at the onset of the Great Depression. As previously mentioned, all American health care professionals were struggling with severe economic hardship. "Dr. Seid used to speak in an amusing fashion about how he'd bring home a sirloin steak with a few potatoes as his fee because [his patients] couldn't give him any money, so the steak fed Seid's family," longtime friend and colleague Morton Abram recalled.[1]

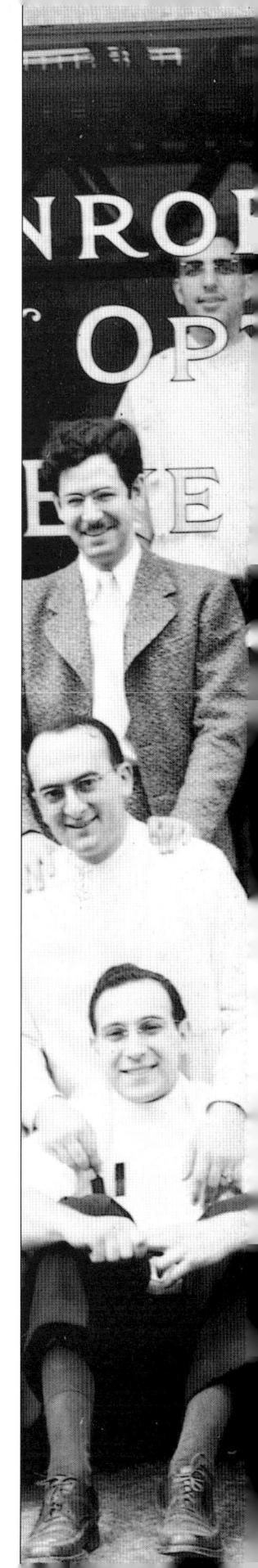

It was time to find another profession. Taking the advice of a close friend, Dr. Samuel Hauser, Dr. Seid decided to go into optometric education. Seid called NICO's Dr. William Needles to request a meeting. He explained to Needles that he planned to start a school of optometry. But Needles wasn't interested in talking with him. As Abram recalled Dr. Seid reminding him on a number of occasions: "If Dr. Needles had really been alert to the situation, and had met with Dr. Seid; [if he] had advised him of all the problems he was going to have in getting the school established — the requirements, etc. including accreditation — Dr. Seid more than likely would have been discouraged and never would have started a school of optometry."[2]

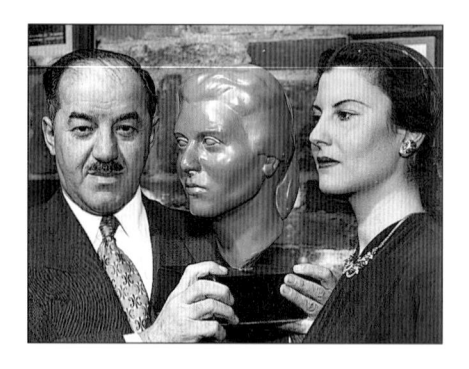

Dr. Needles' early rebuff only reinforced Dr. Seid's determination to establish a new optometric school. And in 1936, he opened the Midwestern College of Optometry. A year later he hired Dr. Carl Shepard from

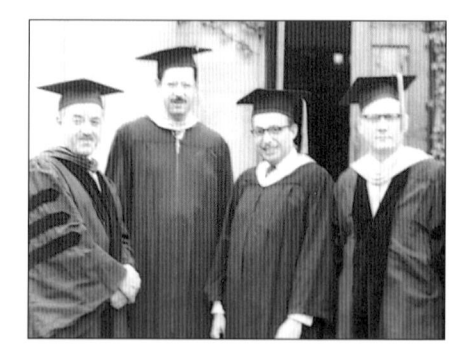

Reuben Seid, Monroe College of Optometry's founder, was an a avid artist. Here, he is pictured with one of his many sculptures and its model.

Graduation day for Eugene Strawn and Hyman Wodis, posing here with Seid and Morton Abram.

Monroe College of Optometry's class of 1942 posed in front of the school located near the Chicago River.

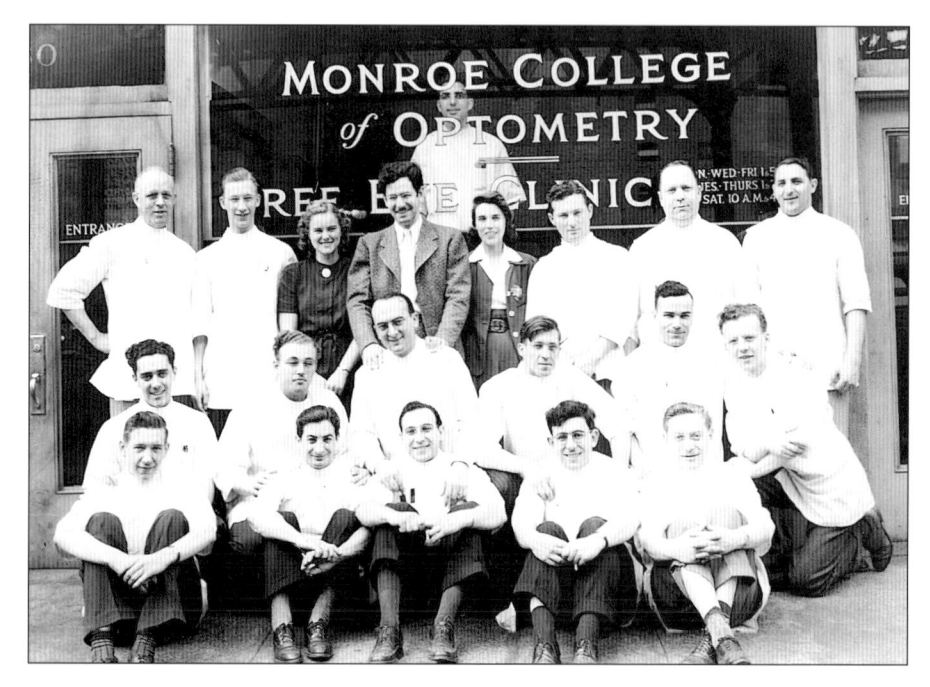

NICO to serve as dean and renamed his school the Monroe College of Optometry (MCO).[3]

Early enrollment was small — less than a dozen students — and because the IBB had not yet accredited the school, graduates were restricted to practice only in Illinois, which already had the nation's largest per capita number of licensed optometrists. In 1941, MCO moved to a 6-story building which had at one time been a poultry market. "They say you could still smell the...chickens down on the ground floor, and it backed up against the Chicago River," Abram remarked. MCO offered a 4-year course which could be completed in three years with summer sessions; tuition was $300 a year.[4]

In 1941, the IBB gave the school's curriculum a Class A rating. Among the school's first diploma recipients were Dr. E.R. Tennant, a recent immigrant from Austria; Dr. Hyman Wodis, who eventually became Chicago College of Optometry's associate dean; and Dr. Eugene Strawn, the 1940 class valedictorian. By 1944, MCO had produced 61 practicing optometrists, not including those in military service.[5]

MCO struggled through the Second World War years for the same reasons as NICO: most young men were drafted into the armed forces. As a recruitment incentive, Seid compressed his 4-year curriculum into a non-stop, 2000-hour/18-month program. Tuition for this program was an astronomical $1000, but the system guaranteed students a quick transition into professional practice. A major scientific development also induced increased enrollment during this period: contact lenses.[6]

CONTACT LENSES, SUNGLASSES AND ENHANCED ETHICS

THE FIRST CONTACT LENSES were simultaneously developed around 1888 by Dr. A. Eugen Fick in Switzerland and Edouard Kalt, a Parisian spectaclemaker. Essentially, both types of contact lenses were thin, fragile, glass lenses which fitted over the eye's entire anterior surface. They were held in place "by atmospheric pressure just as it happens for two wet plates of glass." Obviously, they were expensive to manufacture and dangerous to wear, but prior to the Second World War there were many European and American patients who preferred to risk the hazards for the sake of vanity.[7]

In 1936, the first plastic contact lenses were developed by Dr. William Feinbloom, a Manhattan optometrist. This molded lens was made from a hard plastic resin with a transparent corneal window, but it still fitted over the entire eye. Two years later, John Mullen and Theodore Obrig discovered that hard contact lenses could also be made from polymethyl methacrylate (PMMA) — a shatterproof substance which was (and still is) used in the manufacture of airplane windows. It proved to be a lightweight, transparent material which only minimally reacted with the eye's natural secretions.[8]

Hollywood was quick to popularize contact lenses. They were perfect for changing an actor's eye color for technicolor productions; and were ideal special-effects makeup props for horror and science-fiction movies. In 1940, actor Walter Hampden's blue eyes were changed to brown for his Native American role in the film *Northwest Mounted Police*, thanks to contact lenses. Stage and screen actor Sir Laurence Oliver reputedly owned an entire wardrobe of colored contact lenses which he employed

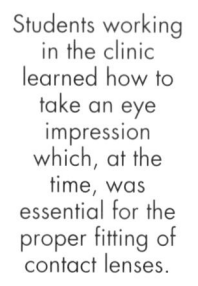

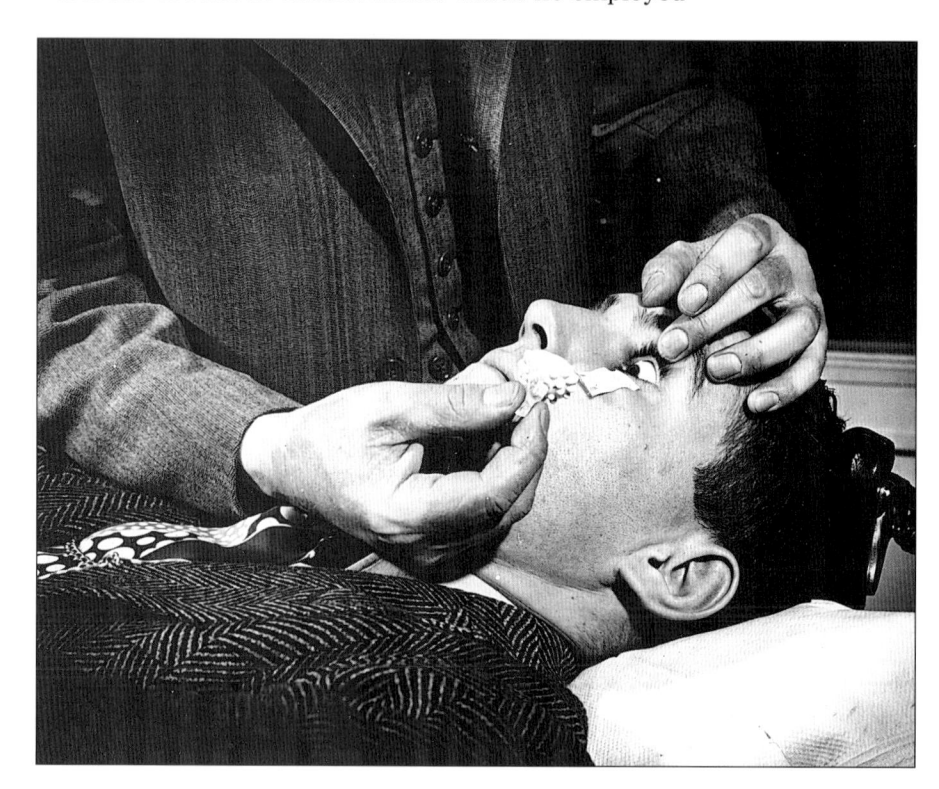

polymethyl methacrylate (PMMA): the chemical term of a polymer resin plastic commercially known as acrylic or plexiglas.

Students working in the clinic learned how to take an eye impression which, at the time, was essential for the proper fitting of contact lenses.

for his various roles. Another celebrity, writer Dorothy Parker, contributed to this eyewear's popularity by reminding women that "men seldom make passes at girls who wear glasses."[9]

But the biggest breakthrough in contact lens development occurred in 1947, when Kevin Tuohy of the Los Angeles-based Solex Laboratories developed the corneal contact lens. By the next year, American optometrists were fitting over 200,000 pairs annually: 3 years before the design was patented.[10]

Another form of eyewear introduced to the public during the 1930s became an even more popular fashion accessory. Sunglasses made with crystal or quartz lenses had been around in China for at least 2000 thousand years. For centuries, Inuit and Siberian tribesmen had been using slit goggles carved from wood or bone to minimize snow blindness caused by the sun's reflective glare. During the sixteenth and seventeenth centuries, Spanish and British scientists also experimented with the use of colored lenses. Later, the Scott, Perry, and Amundsen polar expeditions tested "hi-tech" tinted goggles on their expeditions. But it wasn't until the 1930s, when Polaroid marketed a line of sunglasses, that colored lenses became popular. Besides successfully eliminating glare and blocking some of the damaging effects of direct sunlight on the eyes, sunglasses quickly became a fashion statement thanks to Hollywood celebrities and the movies.[11]

corneal contact lens: a small contact lens which covers only the eye's cornea, not the entire anterior surface.

The Inuit and other Arctic natives wore slit-shaped goggles to block the snow's reflective glare. The Amundsen and Scott South Pole expeditions adapted similar eyewear as well as tinted-glass lenses.

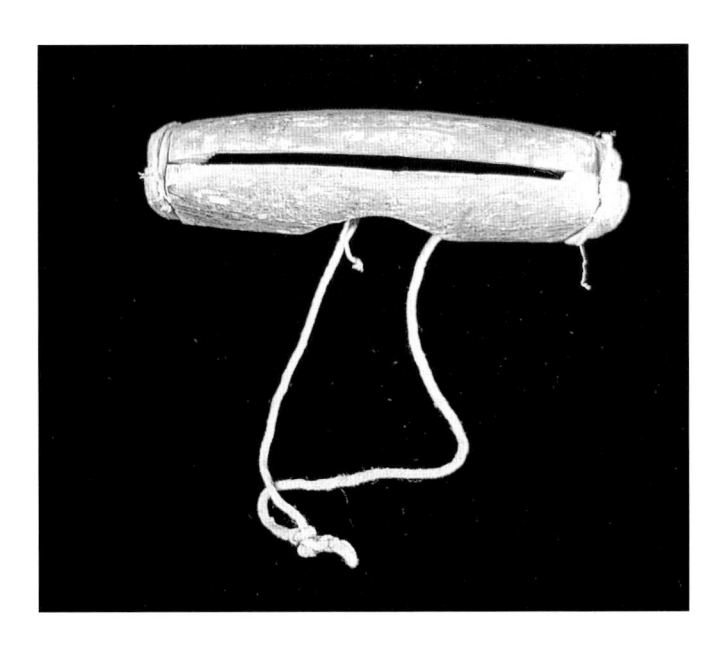

Of the 1347 optometrists serving during the Second World War, there were nearly 300 U.S. Army and Navy officers who provided optometric services. Other practitioners were enlisted men who served as refractionists. Their value was finally recognized and another professional advancement occurred just after war ended, when the federal government created an optometry section in the Army-Navy Medical Corps.[12]

During the war, the AOA enhanced their Code of Ethics. Both AOA members and optometric students graduating after 1944 vowed to practice according to the new oath which more closely resembled the medical profession's Hippocratic Oath. This code covered the basic elements of a fair and competent health care practice. A supplement to this code, added 2 years later, further detailed the practicing optometrist's responsibilities to his patients and his profession.[13]

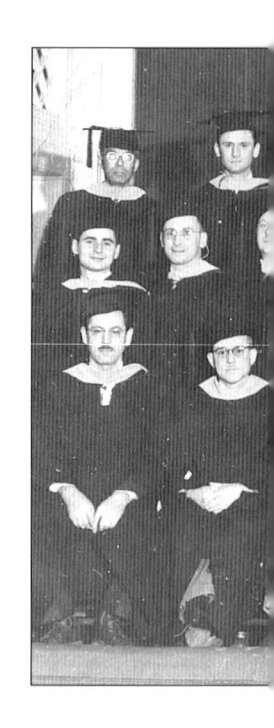

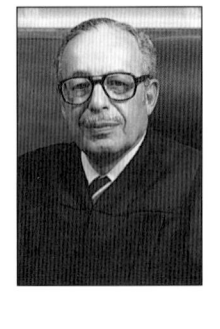

Morton Abram, CCO's business administrator returned to his first profession, law, in later years becoming a Florida judge

ACCREDITATION

AT THE END of the Second World War, Dr. Seid advertised that MCO offered G.I. Bill eligibility. A flood of returning veterans applied: the bill allowed them to explore educational and professional opportunities which might never have been affordable to them otherwise. By 1948, MCO had 500 G.I. Bill enrollees. Schools nationwide were bulging at the seams. But the attrition rate of incoming students was also high — as quickly as they entered many students left, opting for other fields.[14]

When Morton Abram graduated from De Paul University Law School in 1937, "things were rather difficult for a young lawyer starting out with no particular contacts in the legal profession." He accepted a part-time position as an Illinois Division of Rehabilitation field agent, where he first met Dr. Seid. In late 1945, Abram was invited to become MCO's assistant director.[15]

One of Abram's first tasks was to provide enough space for the massive student influx. MCO purchased the 4-story Owen Building on Larrabee Street and an adjacent single-story structure.[16]

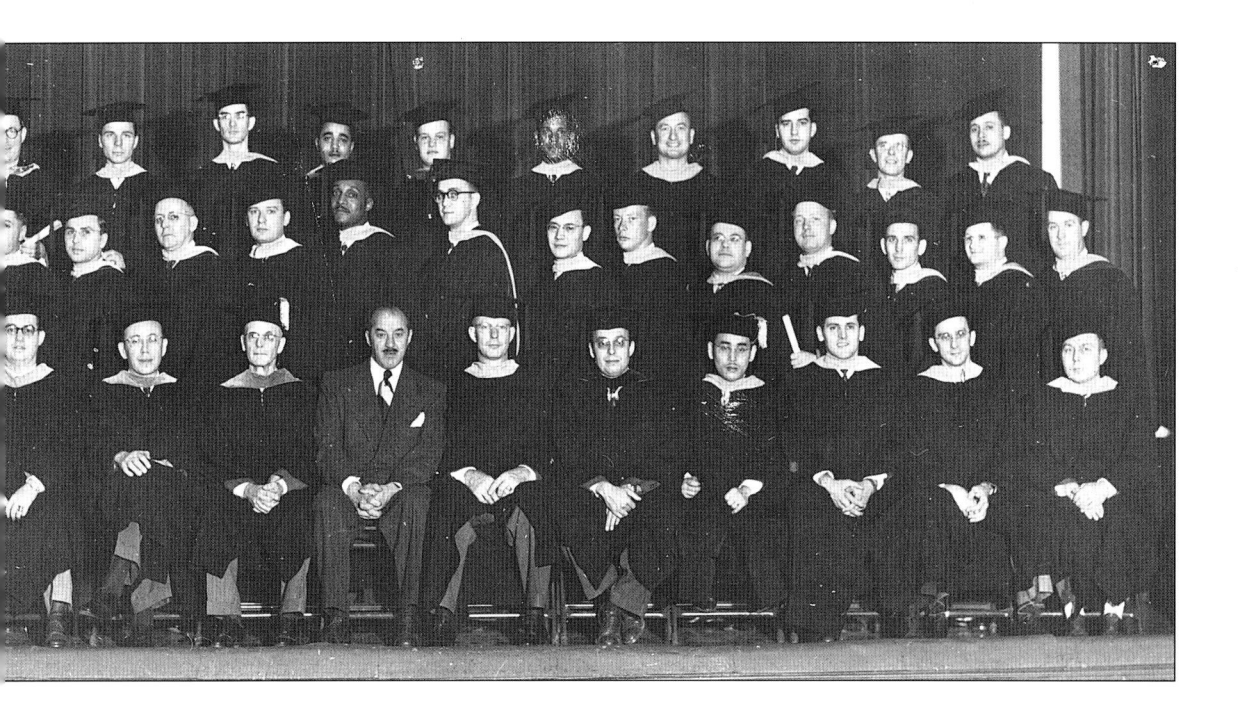

The CCO graduating class and faculty pictured here include: (l-r beginning third from left) Drs. Thaddeus Murroughs, Eugene Tennant, George Hicks, Reuben Seid, unidentified, Morton Abram, and E.S. Takahashi.

But graduates still needed to be licensed outside of Illinois: Abram needed to gain full accreditation for the school. Unfortunately, Seid was considered an outsider by the optometric community. His contacts were members of the medical and vocational education professions. To attain his goal of accreditation, Abram convinced Dr. Seid that they and the school's attorney, Ben Cupple, should attend the 1947 AOA convention in Pittsburgh to meet with the Council on Education, though he knew they would probably be unwelcome guests.[17]

He attempted to contact H. Ward Ewalt, the AOA Council on Education chairman. It was difficult at first, but he persuaded Ewalt — via the AOA's attorney Harold Kohn — that the Council had little to lose by meeting with them. Abram explained to Kohn that MCO had all the best intentions to measure up to the AOA's standards. After the convention's closing banquet, Abram received word that the Council on Education was willing to meet with him in the hotel, and a deal was arranged where the school would be reviewed.[18]

To allow them to begin with a clear slate, Abram changed the school's name to Chicago College of Optometry (CCO); he appointed the school's clinic director, Dr. Hyman S. Wodis, as associate dean in 1949; and filed a Council on Education accreditation application: a 6-

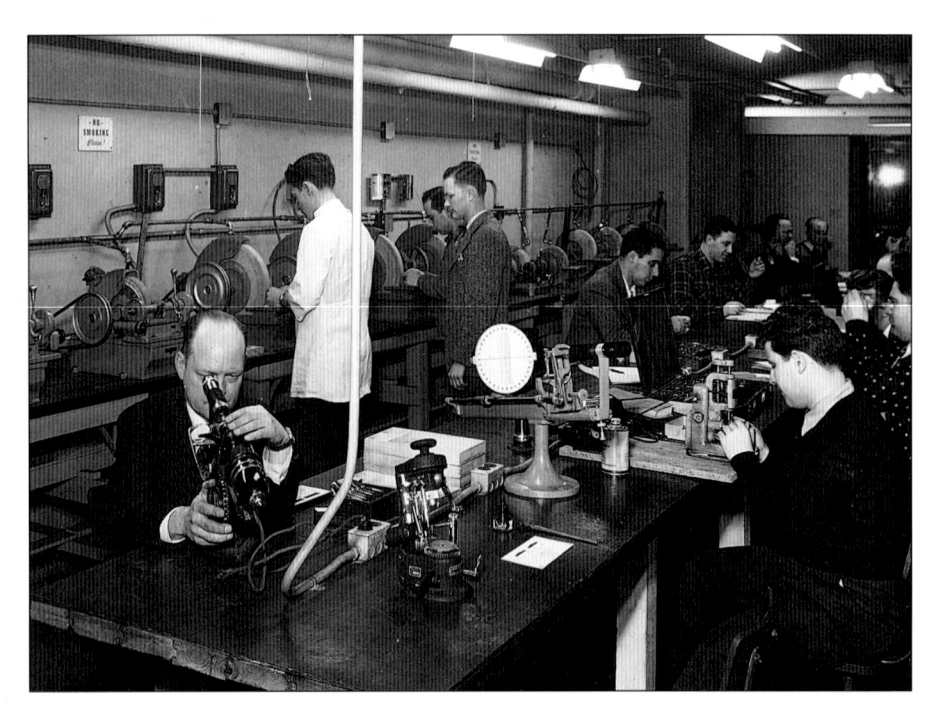

month long process which included submission of statements outlining the school's objectives, academic focus, individual student and graduate development plans, and supporting data schedules. Shortly afterwards, as Abram had been advised, the AOA accreditation committee made an unannounced inspection of the school which included interviewing students and faculty and reviewing the facilities.[19] Several months after this surprise visit, CCO received its provisional accreditation: pending its May 1950 graduation.[20]

CCO established itself with a full 5-year curriculum in 1949: it was one of 3 schools nationwide to do so at that time. Credits for the first 2 years were transferrable from any accredited college or university offering a standard arts and sciences curriculum; while the final 3 years concentrated on optometric science courses and clinical work. Undergraduate tuition was $440 per year, in 1951, and the graduate program cost $550 per year.[21]

The standard optometric curriculum was augmented with courses covering the latest optometric developments and advancements including improved orthoptic techniques, contact lens fitting, occupational vision testing and treatment as well as advanced training techniques to aid patients with reading difficulties.[27]

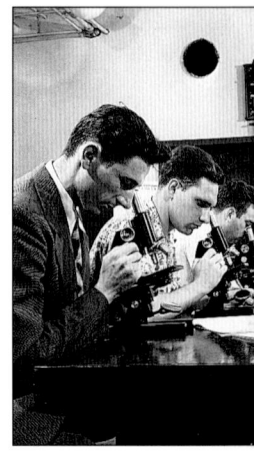

Students trained while serving the needs of north side patients. Lenses and frames were made by students as part of their practical work.

PLATO AND A CHANGING STUDENT BODY

TO KEEP PACE with the rapidly changing technology, Dr. Seid and Morton Abram enlisted an impressive group of optometric scholars as faculty members, including the first African-American optometrist to become a faculty member at an accredited U.S. college, Dr. Junius Brodnax.

Another faculty member, Dr. Eugene Freeman was a NICO graduate and instructor, who also taught philosophy at Illinois Institute of Technology. He had also published a book entitled *Great Ideas of Plato* (1952) which presented a popularized version of the Greek philosopher's works. Freeman additionally combined contact lens research work with an equally successful optometric practice. He became CCO's dean in 1947, while continuing to lecture at Illinois Institute of Technology.[23]

CCO's first clinic administrator was Dr. Ernest S. Takahashi. Under his direction, the facility's 6 departments served 1000-plus patients monthly in 1949. The clinic offered primary optometric examinations, basic medical advice and referral, health care, contact lens laboratory services, visual training, remedial reading, and an eyewear dispensary.[24]

In 1950, Dr. E.R. (Richard) Tennant became the school's clinic administrator. Tennant, who joined CCO's staff immediately after his graduation in 1945, had attended a Viennese medical school until 1938, when the Nazis occupied Austria. Two years later, he escaped the occupied city and immigrated to America. Tennant's 1945 *Introduction to Laboratory Work in Geometrical Optics, Second Edition* syllabus became a CCO standard. When he became clinic administrator, he replaced Dr. Takahashi's "card system" which dictated students' clinical work, with a student-run clinical council program. Dr. Tennant wanted students to "use the clinic as one would use his own office in practice."[25]

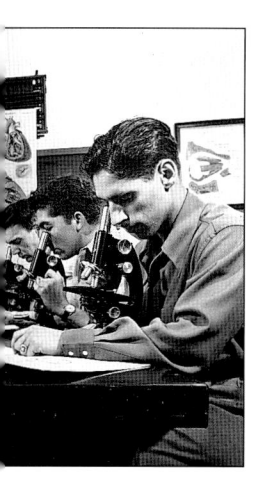

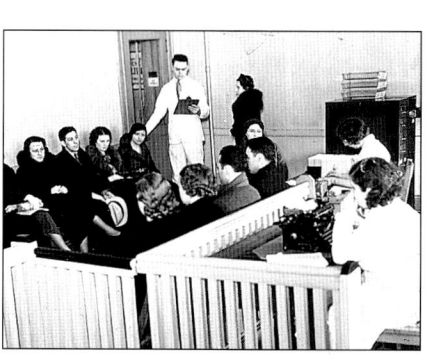

From 1949 through the early 1950s, Dr. Z. John Bruce Schoen headed the optometry department and eventually, headed CCO's graduate program as well. Schoen was a 1932 Ohio State University College of Optometry graduate, with a Masters in psychology from the University of Buffalo, and a doctorate in psychology from the University of Virginia.[26] Under his direction, the school's graduate program, which required students to have both a bachelor's degree and a doctorate in optometry, concentrated primarily on conducting scientific research, and writing formal dissertations.

In 1948, CCO students also took part in the Chicago Strabismus Project, which was jointly sponsored by CCO

CCO's campus was located on Chicago's north side, near Lincoln Park.

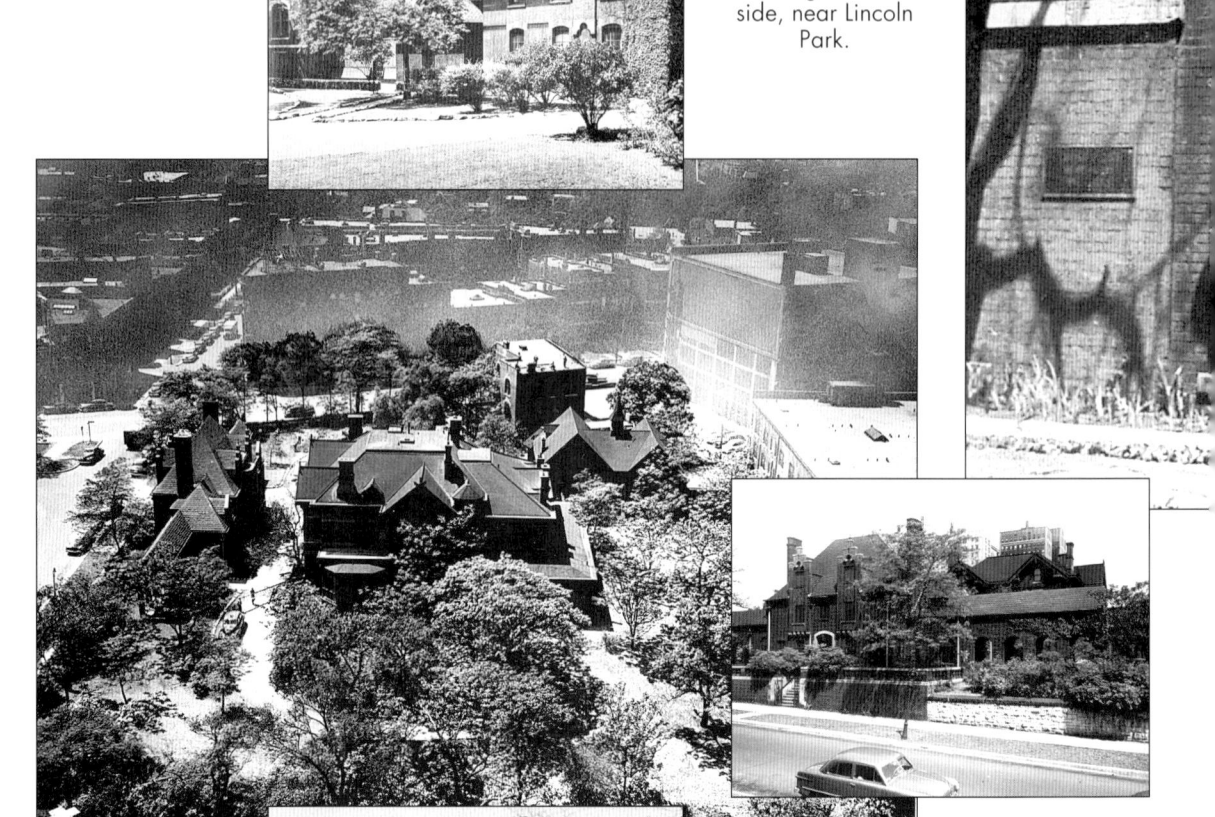

EYES RIGHT

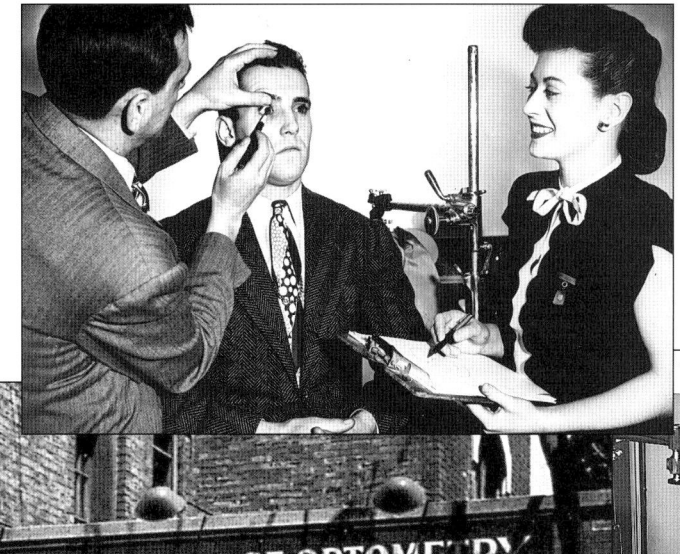

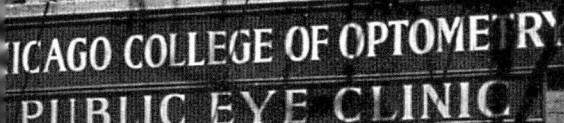

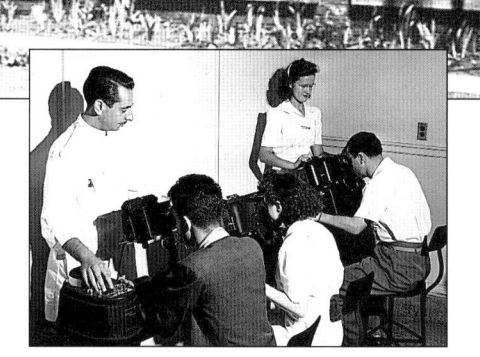

75

TOP: The Dames Club offered students' wives courses geared to preparing young couples for operating a successful private practice together, and held regular teas and luncheons.

CCO's Clinic provided vision training, remedial reading, and other services as well as primary care eye examinations and lens dispensing.

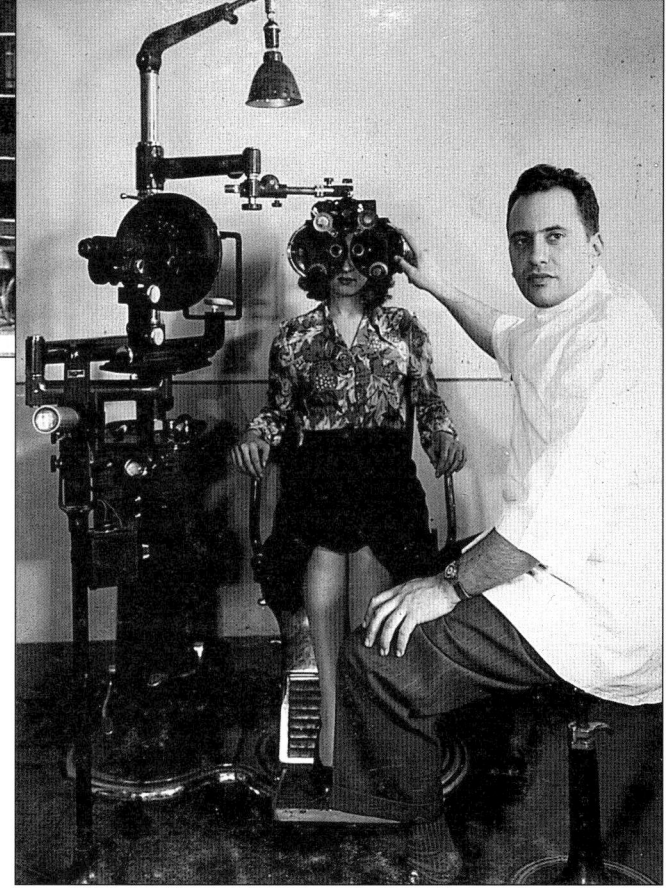

and the Society for Strabismus. The aim of the project was to further the body of knowledge on the causes and treatment of this dysfunction through orthoptic techniques. The Chicago Strabismus Project was directed by Dr. Thaddeus Murroughs, who became CCO's research director in 1950. In addition to his own work on this and other subjects — like a study of eye fatigue, conducted in association with Dr. Leo Manas — Dr. Murroughs established a series of week-long, post-graduate seminars geared for practicing optometrists.[27]

To provide housing for a student body of nearly 800 people, CCO purchased its first dormitory buildings from Illinois State Senator George E. Adams in 1948. The parcel consisted of 5 nineteenth-century brick-and-stone buildings, including the spacious Adams House and equally impressive Evans House which stood together on a verdant landscape near Lincoln Park. Chicago College of Optometry's new campus also included a large public clinic located at the corner of Clark and Belden Streets.

During the 1940 AOA convention, the American Women's Optometric Association was authorized. For years female optometrists had been campaigning for their own association. In schools like NICO, women were also advancing their position as professional practitioners. But unlike NICO, CCO had a relatively small female student population: from 2 to 7 women per class. This was partially due to the fact that the postwar G.I. Bill was not extended to all returning female war veterans. Social attitudes of the time also placed women in the roles of housewives, homemakers, and mothers. The CCO Dames Club — reserved for students' wives — however, offered optometrist's assistant courses (patient record-keeping, assisting during examinations, basic bookkeeping, and general office management). These were valuable skills for 1950s couples who, soon after graduation, started small family practices.[28]

CCO also sponsored an athletic program including The Eyemen basketball team, baseball, tennis, wrestling and fencing teams. The school newspaper, *Eyes-Right* regularly received high ratings from the Associated College Press.[29]

This generation of CCO students was older and more well-traveled than either their predecessors or successors. The 1950 Honor Roll students are prime examples of the CCO student population at that time. Toshimi Ogawa, a 1941 University of Hawaii graduate, had worked as a timekeeper at Pearl Harbor during the war. Earl R. Berkheimer (valedictorian) was a 26-year-old Navy veteran who had previously attended Louisiana Polytechnic Institute. Richard H. Federhar was a 22-year-old, married, Navy veteran who previously had attended the University of Arizona. Williston C. Funk was a 31-year-old, married, Naval Aviation veteran who had previously attended the University of Miami and Butler University. And Bernard Knotts was a 31-year-old, married, Army Medical Corps veteran who had previously attended Glenville State College Their educational and life experiences, prior to entering CCO, generally made these students more adept at concentrating on their studies. It was a determination to succeed in civilian life that also carried over after graduation, when the majority of American optometrists were not only health care providers, they were business owners.[30]

Besides the lucrative funding received from the G.I. Bill, CCO's Eye Clinic generated additional funding through a high volume of examinations and eyewear sales. Both sources contributed greatly to the school's financial stability.

With the success of his school assured, Reuben Seid became involved in the reorganization of Central YMCA College into Roosevelt College (now Roosevelt University). Roosevelt College was designed to be a workingman's institution, where poor but ambitious students could acquire an affordable college education. Under Seid's direction, CCO loaned Roosevelt College $100,000, secured by a mortgage on the historic Adler & Sullivan-designed Auditorium Theater Building. He also did charitable work for the South Shore Hebrew Congregation and the Chicago Art Institute until July of 1951, when Reuben Seid suffered a fatal heart attack. He did not live to witness the ironic turn of events that changed both CCO and NICO's future.[31]

OPTOMETRY
IN AMERICA

78

Color acuity tests are simple, but highly effective tools for determining degrees of color blindness.

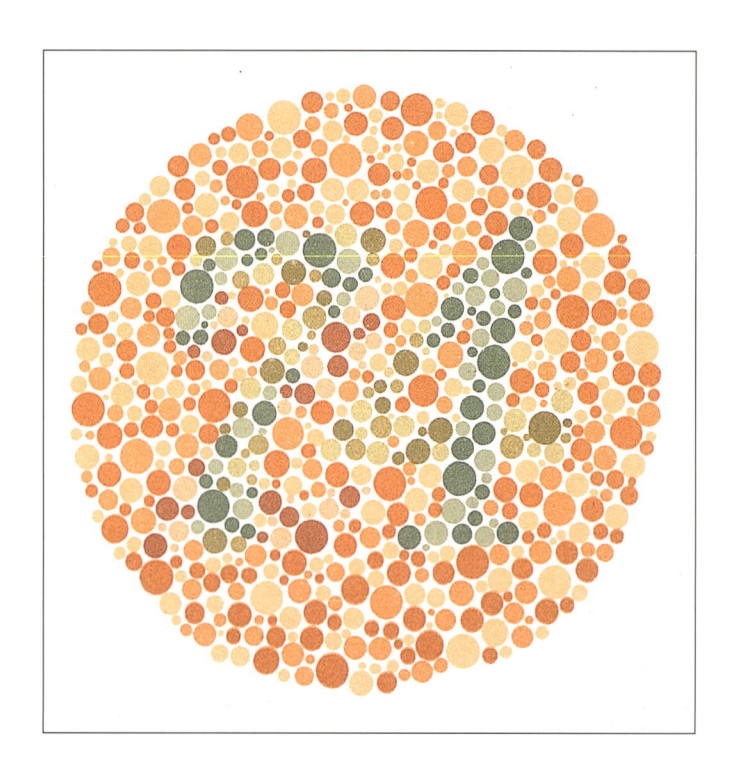

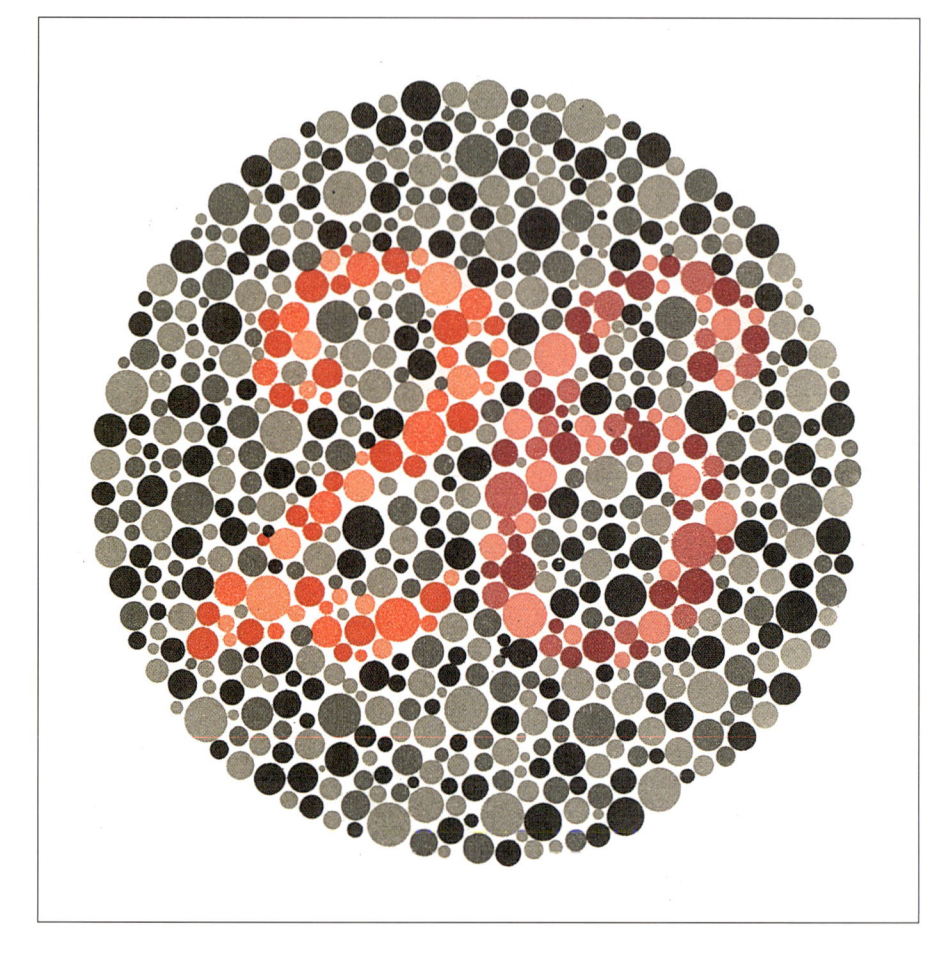

EYES RIGHT

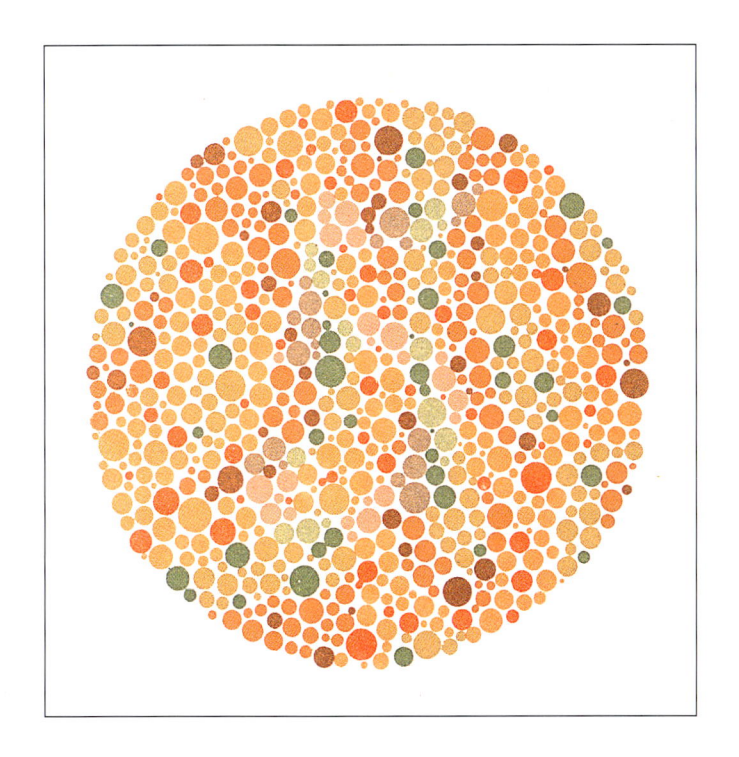

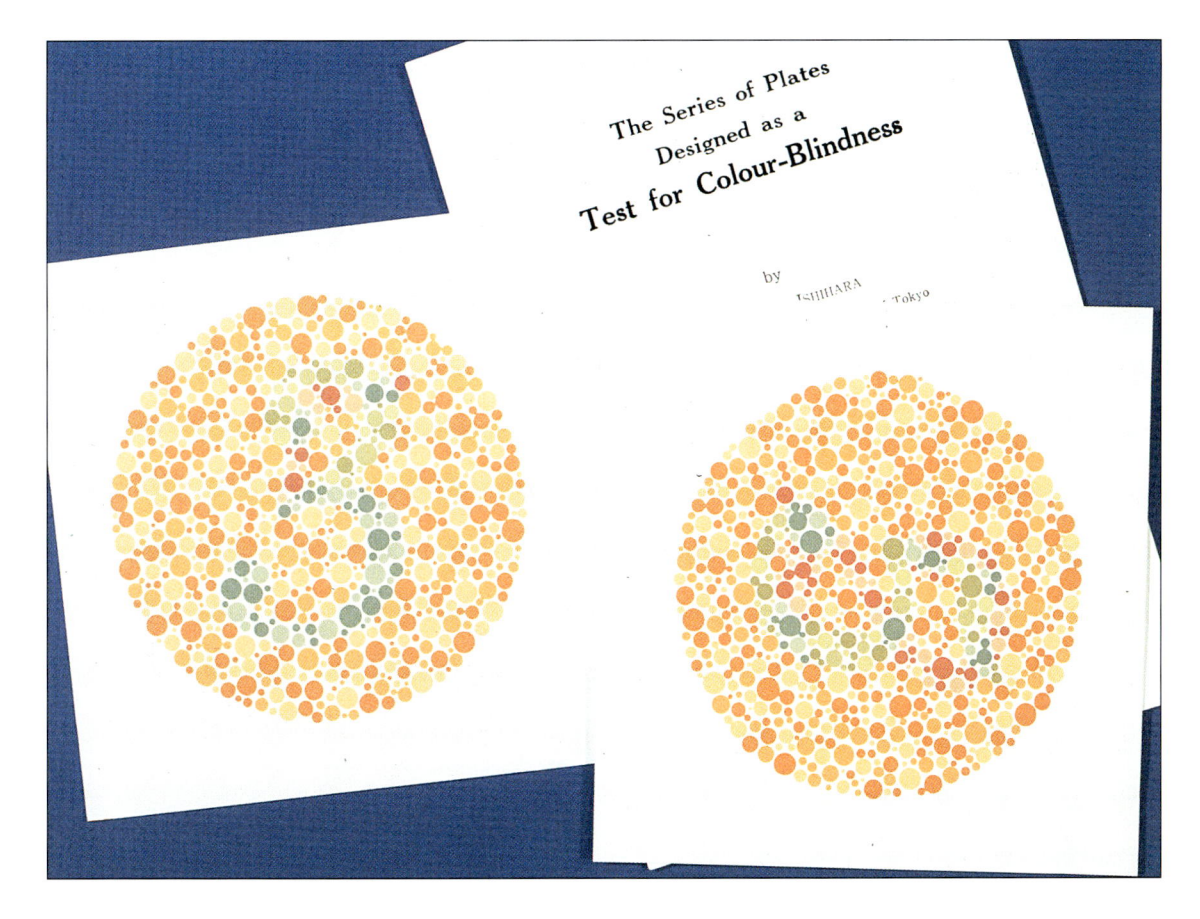

79

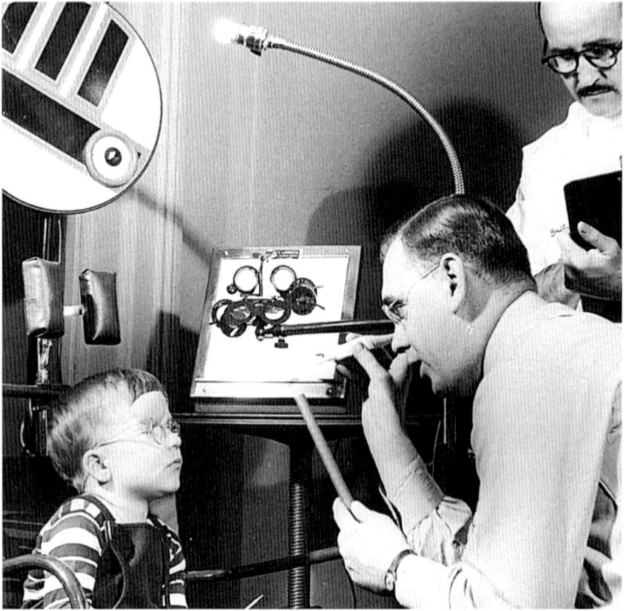

CHAPTER 5

A NEWER WORLD to SEE

THE BIRTH OF ILLINOIS COLLEGE OF OPTOMETRY

A FEATHER IN OUR CAP

EVEN THOUGH STUDENT enrollments hit an all-time high after the Second World War, the number of practicing American optometrists fell, in 1947, to its lowest point in the profession's modern history. There were 4350 students enrolled in the nation's optometric schools, but the post-war boom was over sooner than anyone anticipated. Only 80 new students registered for NICO's 1950 fall session.[1]

To stem this downturn, in 1953, NICO offered student loans and inaugurated an active public relations and marketing program. The Alumni Association, headed by

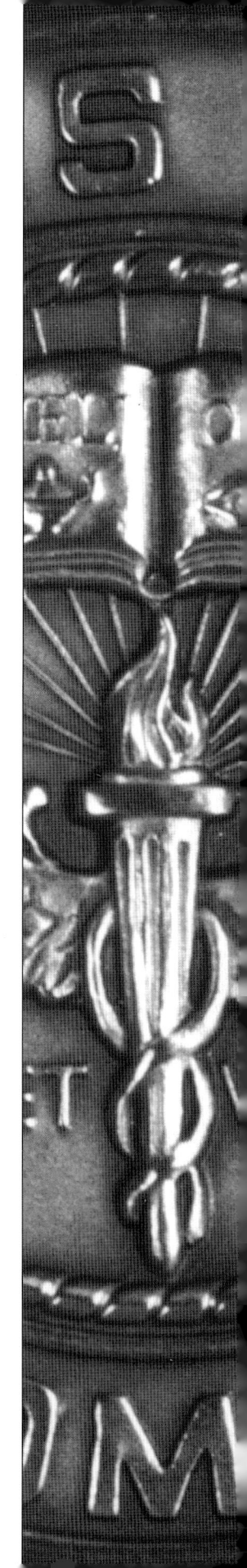

During the 1950s, pediatric vision care was first emphasized in optometric education.

Dr. John Kennedy, hoped to boost enrollment through an alumni selection process. Board member Dr. John Brady appealed to the alumni at a Minneapolis meeting: "How would you like to give the college $1800 without it costing you a cent? Each and every one of you can do that by selecting one student for admission to the next entering class."[2]

But despite their combined efforts, 1952 enrollment was limited to autumn registration. There was not enough demand to continue the school's traditional winter and spring enrollment periods. By 1954 enrollment was becoming a very serious issue at NICO and CCO (where graduation figures had dropped from 480, in 1947, to 94, in 1954).[3]

One factor contributing to both schools' enrollment slump was their location. Chicago's south side and Lincoln Park neighborhoods were rapidly declining. To stem local effects of the 1950s tide of nationwide urban decay, the city of Chicago encouraged several key educational institutions to expand into the city's more run-down areas.

Presbyterian-St. Luke's Hospital and Cook County Hospital, just west of downtown, joined with the University of Illinois Medical School to form a single complex. Both NICO and CCO offered to move to the center, but were refused.[4]

On the south side, the Illinois Institute of Technology (IIT) expanded its campus acreage. Michael Reese Hospital Medical Center followed suit and expanded its borders to meet with 2 new residential middle-income high-rise complexes — Prairie Shores and Lake Meadows.

Morton Abram had become CCO's president after Dr. Seid's death in 1951. He recalled in an interview, "We thought it might be a great feather in our cap if we could build a new institution for ourselves." With Dr. Eugene Freeman's help, Abram contacted IIT's president, John T. Retaliato. Abram hoped to cultivate a close relationship where IIT faculty would teach at CCO, and his students would share IIT's dormitories, cafeteria and commons. But

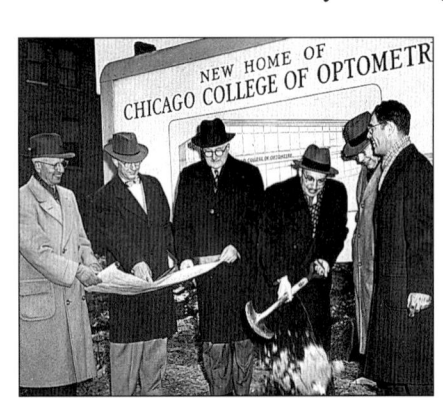

Groundbreaking for CCO's new campus took place one year after the decision was made to move the campus from the north side to a property adjacent to IIT on the south side.

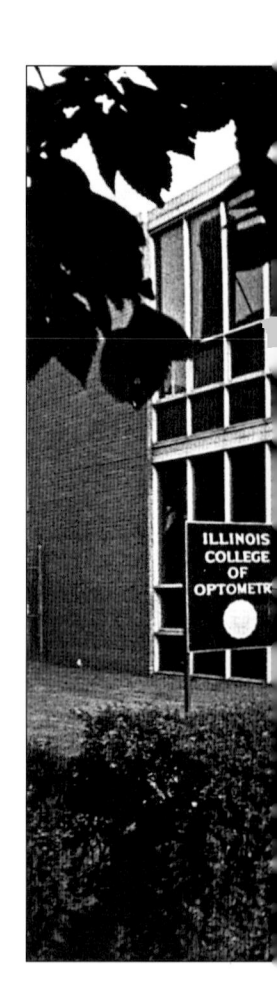

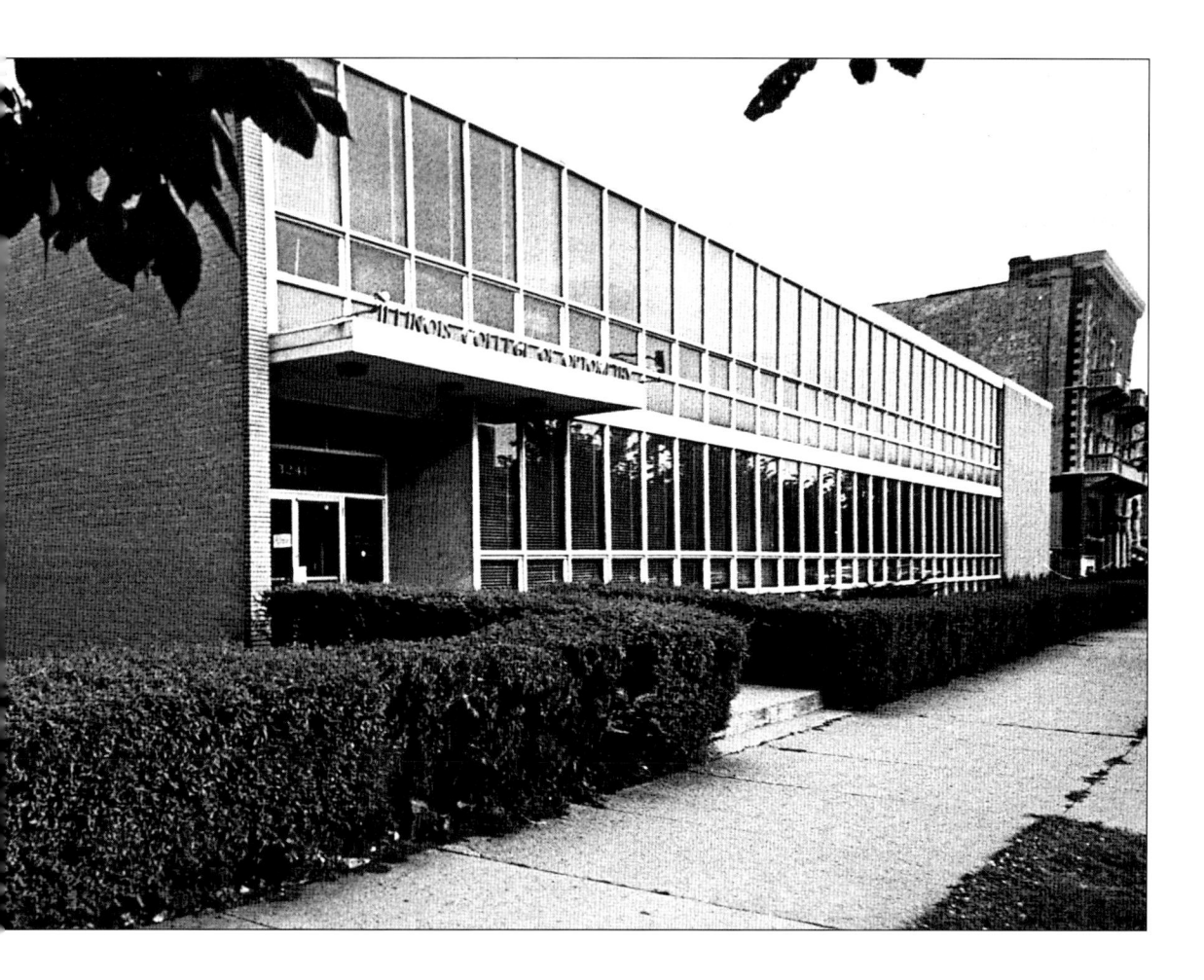

he was told that CCO could not affiliate with a technical institute, but they could build nearby.[5]

With the help of IIT's board chairman, real estate developer Newton Farr, Abram arranged for CCO to purchase an adjacent parcel of land on South Michigan Avenue in 1953. Abram proposed a 20,000 square-foot, 2-story structure designed by the architectural firm of Alexander and Warren Spitz. The architectural design conformed to the Mies van Rohe style found on the IIT campus and the plan was readily approved. Abram also announced the acquisition of a nearby clinic site.[6]

But the groundbreaking ceremony with Farr, Abram, AOA President Dr. James F. Wahl and NICO president Dr. Richard Feinberg did not take place until a year later, on January 29th, 1954. The next fall session was scheduled to commence in the new building and Abram had arranged for CCO students to use IIT's residential, recreational and dining facilities.[7]

The new CCO building reflected the modern lines of IITs Mies van der Rohe designed structures.

Everything was set. Then, on the weekend before classes started, a summer downpour flooded the school's new auditorium. Abram recruited as many helpers as he could find and they frantically bailed water. That Monday, the fall session began on schedule for the schools' 66 incoming students.[8]

AS SIMPLE AS THAT

LOW PROJECTED ENROLLMENTS continued to be Abram's major concern. Soon after the fall session commenced, he called NICO President Dr. Richard Feinberg and asked: "What do you think about the possibilities of merging the two schools?"[9]

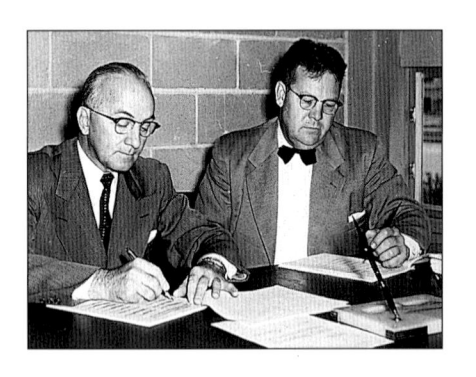

As Abram remembered: "It was just as simple as that. I didn't plan far ahead, I just thought it was the best thing for optometric education and for the profession…Then we had the two boards meet one time at the Medina Hotel, and they spent a whole Sunday talking about the method by which this could be accomplished."[10]

NICO's board chairman, Dr. Glenn H. Moore, and CCO's executive vice-president, Dr. Eugene Strawn, led the discussions. Moore had been instrumental in establishing NICO's status after 1949; and Dr. Strawn, an MCO graduate, had become CCO's executive vice-president after originally being asked to head the Alumni Association earlier that year. Both men concluded that both schools would clearly benefit from a merger.[11]

The schools technically closed their doors on June 9, 1955, reopening together the next day as Illinois College of Optometry (ICO). And even at the outset, there was no doubt the new school was composed of the best its predecessors had to offer. The school's new administration included Dr. Moore as board chairman; Dr. Eugene W. Strawn as president; and Morton Abram as executive vice-president and business manager.[12]

The relatively new CCO building became ICO's home. CCO's North Clark Street clinic — along with a 6-story

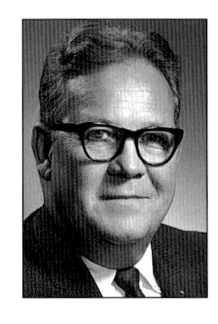

Dr. Glenn H. Moore became ICO's first board chairman after the historic merger.

NICO's Dr. Glenn Moore and CCO's Dr. Eugene Strawn signed the landmark merger between the schools which formed ICO.

Dr. Eugene Strawn, a CCO graduate, became ICO's first president.

apartment building on South Michigan Avenue — served as the ICO Eye Clinic.[13]

ICO's faculty and administrative staff merged the best personnel from both institutions: Dr. Richard Feinberg was appointed dean; Dr. E.R. Tennant became the clinic director; Dr. Hyman Wodis, an MCO graduate and NICO's associate dean became ICO's registrar; and Dr. Walter Yasko, chief of the Northern Illinois Eye Clinic since 1955, was appointed to head the ICO Eye Clinic. Dr. Frederick Kushner had been NICO's dean since 1950, but with the merger, he went into private practice with Dr. John Brady in Iowa. The merged alumni association was headed by Dr. John Kennedy. ICO's combined alumni now represented two-thirds of all American optometrists.[14]

The 1955 fall session registration consisted of 115 new students; and the next month, ICO conferred degrees on its first 16 graduates who were former CCO students.[15]

But increasing enrollment without compromising standards was a challenging task. During the 1950s, the number of lucrative, non-professional jobs available for young men had grown. As mentioned earlier, the social climate of the time encouraged women to stay home rather than pursuing careers or higher education. Even so, the number of female enrollees continued to climb, and there were some notable female students during the decade. For example, Second Lieutenant Freda J. Slaymaker, a 1956 ICO graduate, became the first female U.S. Army optometrist in 1961.[16]

The total 1958 enrollment at all American optometric colleges fell to a low of 1136 students: fewer than 90 students were enrolled at ICO. But academic institutions nationwide were very aware of the post-war baby boom and began planning ahead rather than dwelling on the existing small enrollments. The United States population had increased greatly after the Korean War, and educators knew they would soon have a great influx.[17]

Dr. Frederick Kushner was appointed as ICO's Alumni Association president, in 1956, while continuing with his private practice. Through his "Kushner's Korner" columns in the *ICO Newsletter*, he kept the alumni informed about their peers and asked that every member "should find at least ONE student for next year. Every state should set up a scholarship." Without additional

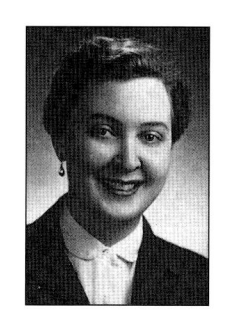

Dr. Freda J. Slaymaker, a 1956 ICO graduate, became the first female U.S. Army optometrist in 1961.

staff, he set about the job of uniting alumni to aid their school.[18]

Dr. Kushner's appeals worked. ICO had 80 new enrollees for the 1961 fall session. And in 1962, another 89 students signed on, including Philip Needles (Dr. Richard Needles' son) and David DeVere (son of former AOA President and NICO alumnus, Dr. Paul N. DeVere).[19]

The next year, ICO promoted optometric career opportunities in a series of public service radio announcements played on 137 midwestern radio stations. The initial response was favorable. Enrollment climbed and the promotional program was soon broadcast nationwide.[20]

Between 1961 and 1968, the average first-year ICO student still scored in the top 25 percent on Optometric College Aptitude Tests (OCAT), and a third of all enrollees already had bachelor's degrees. To fill in the gaps left by a temporary enrollment decrease, and to prepare for the coming projected influx, ICO launched a major fundraising campaign in 1961 — soliciting corporate, foundation and private financial support to create an endowment fund to support research, to construct new facilities, and to increase the faculty.[21]

FEDERAL ACCEPTANCE AND ASSISTANCE

OPTOMETRY WAS ACCORDED further governmental and health care industry acceptance when it was included in the federal Health Professions Educational Assistance Act of 1963, signed by President John F. Kennedy. This bill allowed optometric colleges to take advantage of new federal matching funds granted to health care-oriented educational institutions.[22]

The AOA's Department of National Affairs reported, in 1968, that numerous federal agencies were employing full-time and consulting optometrists for health care programs including: the Civil Service Commission, the Veterans Administration, the Indian Health Service, the Department of Defense, the Department of Health, Education and Welfare (HEW), the Public Health Service, the Department of Transportation, the General Services

Administration, and the Office of Equal Opportunity (OEO).[23]

The OEO and HEW launched roughly 150 neighborhood health centers in 1967 as part of a federal program sponsored by Senator Edward M. Kennedy. Half of these centers provided optometric services. The various military service branches along with federal and state public assistance departments found optometry an essential service in their "one-stop" health care programs. Almost half of the nation's medical schools also helped to develop and staff these centers with physicians to work side-by-side with the optometrists. And many hospitals contributed additional programs.[24]

President Kennedy's administration had made community-based medical services with federal funding for community clinics and hospital aid a political priority during the 1960 Congress. But it wasn't until President Lyndon B. Johnson took office that the Medicare and Medicaid programs gained enough house votes to be passed. (Medicaid is part of the state-controlled public assistance system, unlike Medicare, which is governed by the Social Security Administration). This federally-funded state program guaranteed the nation's poor access to adequate health care. Optometry was included in the government's 1965 list of Medicaid services.[25]

Federally-funded scholarship and research programs increased student opportunities in the early days of ICO.

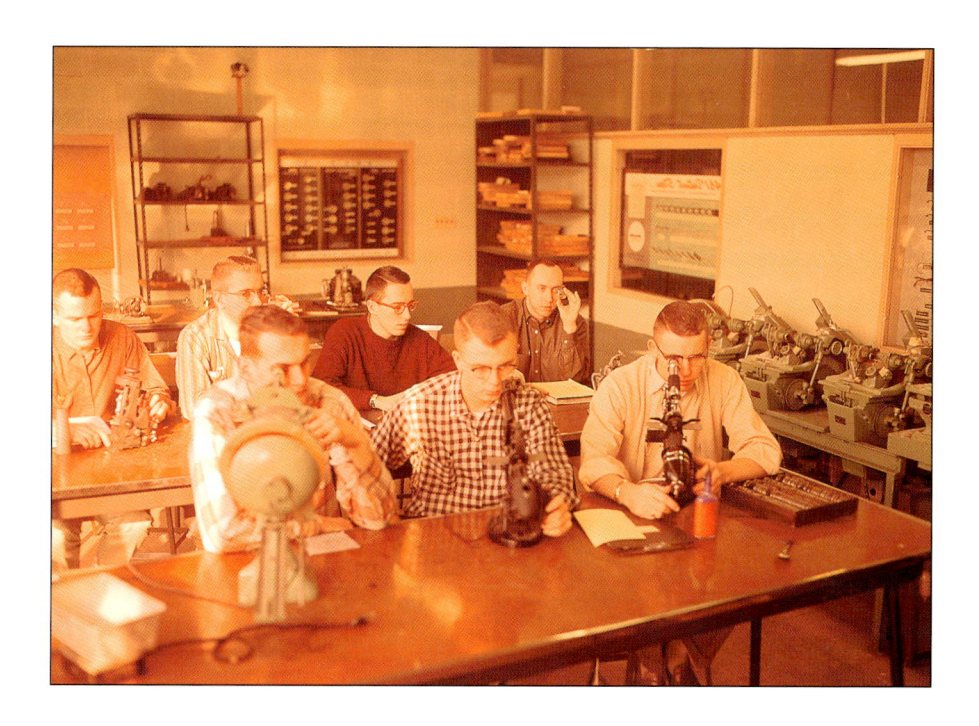

Other newly-created federal aid programs to educational institutions underwrote much of ICO's 1960s and 1970s development. Federally-funded student loans, scholarships, and basic improvement grants, combined with increased enrollment, contributed to ICO's — and almost every educational institutions' — financial stability. From the inception of the 1961 alumni endowment drive, it was also hoped that funding would "come from participation, and total assets of the foundation will be increased primarily through the support and cooperation of the alumni of ICO."[26]

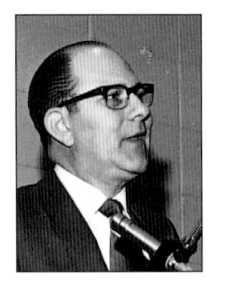

Working along with Dr. Kushner in campaigning for alumni support was Dr. C.K. Hill, a 1949 NICO graduate, who proved to be a champion alumni fund-raiser. He converted one room of his home, in 1961, into an ICO alumni office. Together, they planned a major fund drive, asking each alumnus to authorize his optical supplier to add $10 monthly to his bill and send that money to the alumni office. Hill also spent 3 years assembling ICO's first alumni roster.[27]

ICO relied heavily on IIT student housing, library, and cafeteria services. As both ICO and IIT's student enrollments increased, this became a problem. In May 1964, ground was broken for Brady Hall (named after former board chairman the late Dr. John J. Brady), a 3-story dormitory to house 170 unmarried male students. One of the project's prominent supporters was Combined American Insurance Company and its affiliates which were owned by Chicago insurance mogul and motivational book author W. Clement Stone. (Dr. Hill had brought ICO's needs to Stone's attention.) Remaining funds came from Alumni Association pledges and a 1964 Health Professions Educational Assistance Act matching grant.[28]

When Brady Hall was dedicated on May 30th 1965, ground was also broken for a clinic wing. Alumni sup-

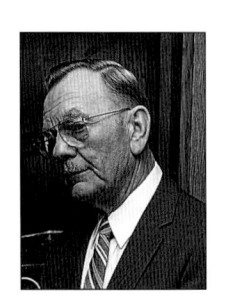

Dr. C.K. Hill worked with Dr. Fred Kushner to champion the Alumni fund drives that financed many of ICO's programs.

Brady Hall's dedication ceremony was paired with the groundbreaking for further expansion of the ICO campus.

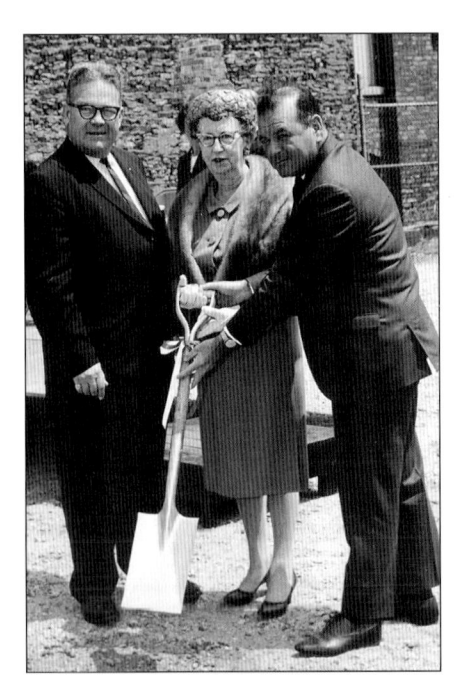

Attending the 1968 cornerstone laying ceremony were (from left to right) Dr. Walter S. Yasko, Ms. Lillian Licheniack, Drs. Jess Goroshow, Alfred A. Rosenbloom, Jr., Eugene Strawn, Hyman Wodis, and Mr. Hugh Ashby.

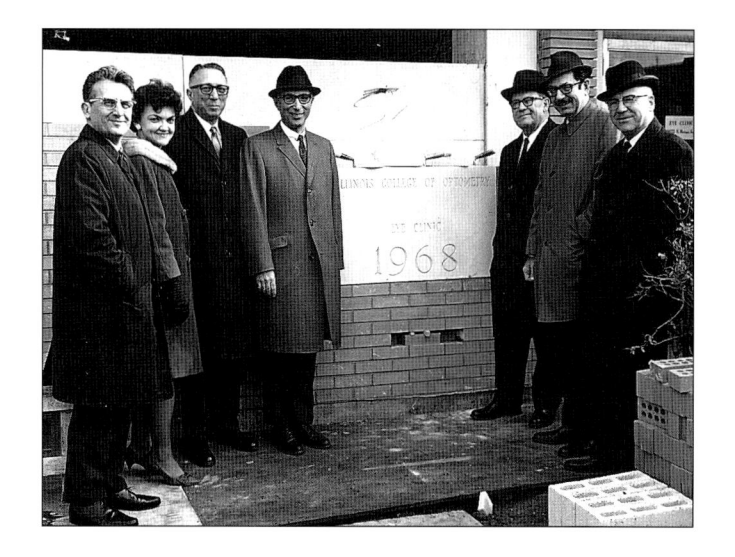

A NEWER WORLD TO SEE

89

port, further federal matching grants, and mortgaging funded more improvements including an instructional wing with additional library, classroom, research, and office space; another residence hall; and a married students' apartment building.[29]

Even though ICO's building plans were approved by the city's zoning and urban renewal agencies, they encountered a roadblock with the Department of Streets and Sanitation. The department had commenced with their own plans to widen Michigan Avenue to a 4-lane, 150-foot wide parkway just north of 31st Street.[30]

"I pointed out," Strawn wrote in an article, "that if the project went forward…Michigan Avenue would run down the center of our main hallway in our college building. …We were at that time negotiating…a dormitory adhering to the same frontage line, and that if these plans could not be altered or changed or revised, I would have to notify the board of trustees with a likely prospect of liquidating our holdings in this area and moving to the suburbs." It took nearly a year to reach the final resolution, allowing ICO to develop their plans in June of 1968.[31]

Dr. Strawn and the contractors condensed the original 2-phase plan into a single phase; and by the 1969 fall session, the new Illinois Eye Institute and the Alumni Memorial Instructional Wing were completed. The buildings were dedicated in October, "to the task of providing the finest education for optometrists…so they in turn may take care of the vision care for the citizens of this great city of Chicago." [32]

CHANGES IN ATTITUDE AND CURRICULUM

DURING THE LATE 1950s and early 1960s, "we began to assemble information that would eventually culminate in our accreditation with the North Central Association of Colleges and Secondary Schools," Strawn stated in his dedication speech. He further added: "This is unique because we are the first and only independent health care college in the region that has been accredited by the North Central Association."[33]

This period was also a career highlight for Dr. Alfred A. Rosenbloom, Jr., who was appointed dean in 1956. Rosenbloom was a Phi Beta Kappa Pennsylvania State College graduate had received his doctorate from NICO, and had been awarded one of the first American Optometric Foundation fellowships. He had also earned a University of Chicago masters degree in higher education for his thesis on *The Relationship of Certain Visual Abilities to Achievement in Reading at the Elementary Grade Level*. Rosenbloom was a great believer in the concept that optometry should be the primary subject taught to optometric students — just like his predecessor Dr. William Needles.[34]

But in 1966, tests revealed that an alarming number of first-year students needed additional liberal arts work. This problem affected many American higher-education institutions. Elementary and secondary schools had been so taxed by the baby boom that some college-bound students were deficient in basic skills like reading, language arts, communications, and mathematics. Some optometric educators argued that students needed more liberal arts and science pre-requisites, while others argued that the profession itself had grown more complex and required an additional year of scientific coursework. As many optometric schools did at that time, ICO added first-year courses like "Communication Skills for the Professional Man" and "Methods of Science" to appease both camps. However, they did not add courses in foreign languages, history or philosophy as other institutions had done.[35]

The 1960s was a radical period, filled with national civil unrest and international military escalation. But it was also

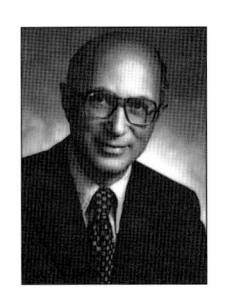

Dr. Alfred A. Rosenbloom, Jr. became ICO's dean in 1956.

DPAs: diagnostic pharmaceutical agents such as anesthetics, mydriatics, cycloplegics, and miotics which are used to anesthetize the eye's sensitivity to touch or to dilate the eyes for interior observation during a patient examination.

a time when optometry's professional standing among other health care disciplines — and with the public — was being affirmed by the legal and academic recognition of the Doctor of Optometry (O.D.) degree which is equivalent to medical and dental doctorates. By the mid-1960s, the O.D. degree was attainable at all of the nation's optometric educational institutions. (Though a bachelor's degree was preferred, a minimum of 3 years of undergraduate pre-optometric education with similar requisites to those found in medicine and dentistry was and is required.) A requirement of 800 additional clinical training hours was also added to the ICO curriculum, and fourth-year students now served in the clinic as both examiners and junior staff instructors.[36]

In 1971, the state of Rhode Island enacted legislation permitting optometrists to use diagnostic pharmaceutical agents (DPAs). (Use of these drugs was previously relegated to ophthalmologists. In the profession's early history, optometrists strongly objected to their use in examinations, but increased awareness of a variety of ocular pathologies made their use critical to thorough and objective vision testing.) To answer this call for additional education, a third year of special procedures lab work was added to supplement the existing clinical internship. Ophthalmic pharmacology, developmental psychology, developmental vision, public and community health optometry, and additional strabismus-amblyopia study were added to the curriculum. A new learning resources department was established to broaden the range of available learning materials: closed-circuit television cameras in selected lecture, lab, and clinical areas allowed in-house film, audio, and video tapes to be developed.[37]

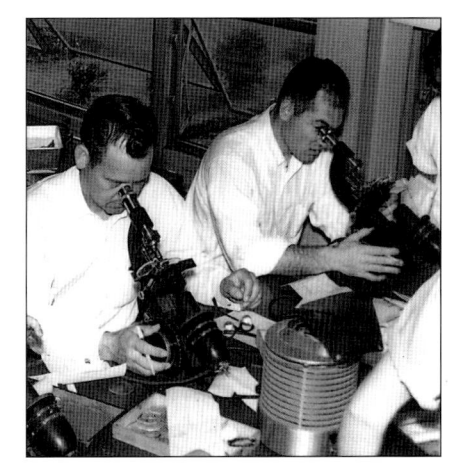

Meanwhile, the AOA's numerous committees were also involved in refining the profession. They were lobbying for legislation that would make optometric services available to veterans on an out-patient basis (Bill H.D. 7966). They revised the AOA *Manual on Drive Vision Tests* which was implemented nationwide by state motor

Students in ICO's lensometry lab learned how to grind, polish and measure lenses.

vehicle departments. Dr. Frederick Kushner was chairman of the AOA's Committee on Practice Management which developed new public education materials for distribution in practitioners' offices and in schools. His committee also revised the practice management kit and the service pricing booklet *Professional Optometric Fees*.[38]

THE MANAS MAZE AND EYE INSTITUTE EXPANSION

BEGINNING IN 1958, Dr. Rosenbloom concentrated his efforts on a student externship program which was intended to provide students with hands-on field experience in a variety of off-campus settings. William A. Johnson's externship is one example of this program's value. The 1966 student extern worked at the Great Lakes U.S. Naval Hospital under the supervision of Rear Admiral J. W. Albrittain, where he "participated in refracting and dispensing services and observed all of the activities of the diversified optometric-ophthalmological clinic." Supported by the alumni association, students worked during vacation periods in private and government practices, many of which were owned and operated by alumni.[39]

Dr. Rosenbloom, along with Drs. Leo Manas, Paul F. Shulman, and others, conducted both on- and off-campus continuing education courses as visual training, developmental vision, and other areas of the optometric practice advanced in scope.[40] By December 1956, contractors had completed the remodeling of the 20,000 square foot, 3-story ICO Eye Clinic. (Mayor Richard J. Daley was the guest speaker at the dedication ceremonies.) The new clinic had 25 refracting rooms, outfitted with the latest optometric equipment. The 1960 alumni donors, in another fund-raising drive, helped furnish and equip examination rooms. By autumn, 3 fully-equipped rooms were installed. And the next year, the South Carolina Alumni Chapter donated an additional room. Dr. Yasko supervised student clinicians in this new

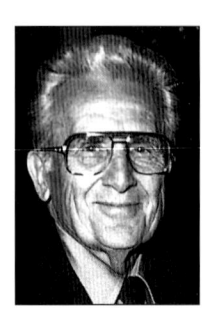

Heading the ICO Eye Clinic was Dr. Walter Yasko, who had previously directed ICO's Northern Illinois Eye Institute.

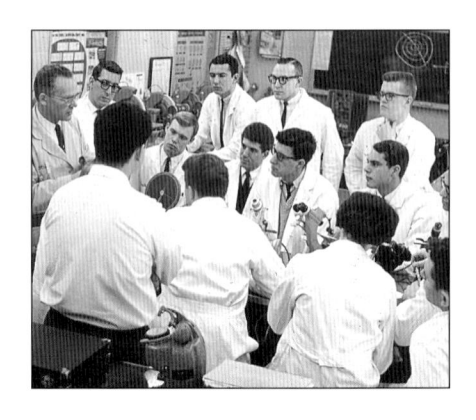

ICO students attending classes in new, state-of-the-art facilities.

setting as they each attended at least 150 patients annually.[41]

Nine years later, a 2-story clinic extension was constructed with 40 additional examination rooms, plus space for instruction and practical application of contact lenses, visual training and other services. Clinicians also continued to provide services at the Robert R. McCormick Boys Club on Chicago's north side. Thanks to an annual donation from W. Clement Stone, each year, an ICO graduate was awarded a $6000 year-long residency at the Boys Club.[42]

Optometry took another step forward thanks to the work of NICO graduate and author of the *Visual Analysis Handbook* (1953) Dr. Leo Manas, who specialized in visual training and had worked with Dr. Thaddeus Murroughs in strabismus research. Working as an optometry professor in ICO's visual training department, Manas invented the Manas Maze (also known as the ICO Maze), in 1959, after a visit from an electronics engineer whose daughters needed visual training. The engineer offered to combine his expertise with Manas' optometric knowledge to produce a testing and training device for his daughters' use. Their collaboration was a success. The maze is not only used in evaluating the projection and fixation ability of the monocular case; or for evaluating suppression patterns under dynamic conditions. It has also proved to be an invaluable training device for pediatric suppression cases, as well as in pediatric arm-hand and eye performance training. Ten years after its invention, Manas Maze units with with additional form templates were first marketed outside of the school, for $155 each. Dr. Manas donated his patent rights to the school to fund further research work into visual training devices. (The Manas Maze was later refined by Manas' student and colleague, Dr. John Roggenkamp.)[43]

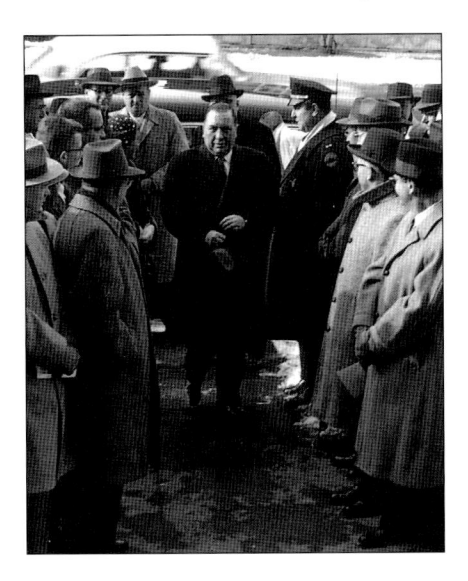

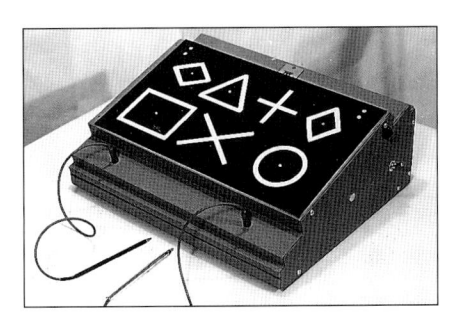

Chicago's mayor Richard J. Daley attended the 1956 dedication ceremony.

The Manas Maze was a vision training apparatus developed at the school by Dr. Leo Manas (below) in the 1950s.

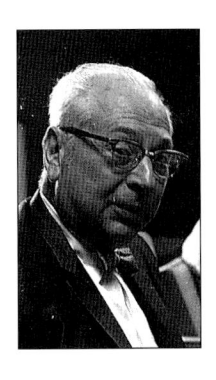

AFFIRMATIVE ACTION AND FURTHER AFFILIATIONS

ESTABLISHING ICO had taken its toll on Dr. Strawn, and in 1969, he appointed ICO registrar, Dr. Jess E. Goroshow, to the new post of assistant to the president. As overall administrative assistant, Goroshow handled student finances and special services, government grants, and reports. Two years later, Dr. Strawn was attending an American Academy of Optometry meeting in Toronto, when he succumbed to a heart attack.[44]

Board chairman Dr. O.W. Weinstein became interim president as the board committee searched for Strawn's replacement. In March 1972, Dr. Rosenbloom was chosen to be the school's president. Maintaining his post as dean, Rosenbloom became the first ICO President to be formally inaugurated. (During the hectic days of the merger, no ceremony had accompanied Strawn's appointment.)[45]

Before his untimely death, Strawn had planned ICO's Centennial (May 30-June 4, 1972) based on the theme "A Newer World To See." Luci Johnson Nugent, daughter of former President Lyndon B. Johnson, was named the Centennial's Honorary Chairman. As a child she had attended the best schools and worked hard, but her academic performance had been poor. The Johnsons were extremely concerned until Luci's eyes were examined: the optometrist detected vision problems and corrected them. As an adult and mother, Mrs. Nugent was acutely aware of "the heartache that inadequate visual performance can bring a child." She served as Honorary Chairman of Volunteers for Vision: a national organization committed to improved pediatric vision care. She was also active with the AOA's Women's Auxiliary in the Project Head Start Program on the War on Poverty.[46]

At the inauguration, Rosenbloom pledged new directions for the college. He promised to broaden and diversify the student body; to meet the new demands for curriculum development; encourage further involvement in scholarly pursuits; and to provide new resources and opportunities for off-campus interdisciplinary training.[47]

More African-American, Hispanic-American, Native-American, Asian-American, and female students enrolled in the early 1970s than ever before. Vietnam War veterans also helped to increase enrollment to 442 students. ICO obtained a federal Minority Recruitment grant and hired an experienced educational administrator, Oliver Slaughter, to manage the program along with an ICO clinical instructor, Dr. Carl Ellis.[48]

ICO also kicked-off a "Promise to Go Back" scholarship which funded students who pledged to work in minority neighborhoods — where their services were desperately needed — after graduation. The first recipient was Carletta Boyd, a Chicago native who planned to open a south side practice.[49]

The AOA's Women's Auxiliary as well as many state and local organizations were already providing Head Start and Upward Bound programs with visual screening services. The national Job Corps and Neighborhood Youth Corps programs also gave optometrists opportunities to provide much needed vision care in depressed areas with equipment supplied by the Lions Club, the Corps themselves, and participating optical laboratories.[50]

Dr. Peter Nelson and some of his ICO students independently launched the Vision Project in 1972 to bring optometric services to underprivileged residents of Chicago's Inner City. Equipment for the project was donated by alumni and other school supporters. Vision screenings commenced at the Albizu Campos Center for the People's Health and were later extended to the Benito Juarez Clinic and the Erie House Clinic. Patients needing additional care were referred to the Illinois Eye Institute or the Northwestern University Medical School Department of Ophthalmology.[51]

ICO continued the affiliated clinic work at the McCormick Boys Club and expanded its program to include the Gilchrust-Marchman Rehabilitation Center of the Easter Seal Society of Metropolitan Chicago, Inc., the

ICO's Centennial seal proudly commemorated the merger of two great optometric institutions and 100 years of optometric education.

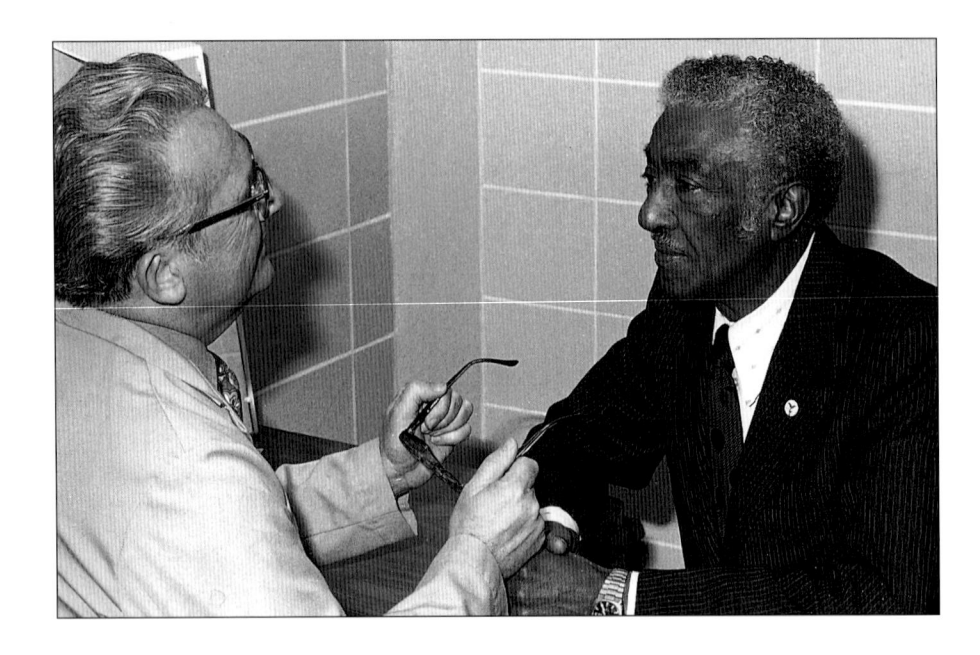

Dr. Walter Yasko (left) fitting U.S. Congressman Ralph Metcalfe for a pair of glasses during visit to ICO's clinic.

Maryville Academy, and the U.S. Government Medical Center in Hines, Illinois. Later affiliations included the Illinois Visually Handicapped Institute, the Japanese/American Service Committee, LaPaz Child Development Center, and the Little City Eye Clinic.[52]

Affirmative action was being instituted in the nation's educational system. But even before the minority recruitment project was established and federal action made it mandatory, ICO was honored by the National Optometric Association (NOA), in 1973, for its "true commitment to social consciousness." Dr. C. Clayton Powell, NOA President, noted at the award ceremony that ICO had the nation's largest, most successful minority recruitment program at that time.[53]

The students' social commitment also stretched far beyond the local area. Fourth-year students David Duryea, Neil Einhorn, James Kirchner, and Don Vanderfelz joined a 1977 Indiana University student team of 9 people in Haiti to take part in the Volunteer Optometric Services to Humanity (VOSH) program. Vanfeltz commented in an interview, "You get to help a lot of patients who otherwise wouldn't have received any eye care." Over the course of 4 days, the student team worked with 18 optometrists, examining 4566 patients, dispensing nearly 3000 prescriptions and fitting 8 prosthetic eyes. "It's a learning experience we can't duplicate at the college," Duryea reported. "You get to see a lot of pathology in a short time."[58] Arranged by

ICO trustee Dr. Walter Marshall, this and future trips opened the doors for ICO students and faculty to partake in VOSH programs in the Caribbean, Central, and South America.[54]

ICO students and faculty also dispensed vital eye care through the school's long-standing affiliation with the Chicago Lighthouse for the Blind: a rehabilitation and training center for patients who are classified as legally blind.

The ICO Eye Clinic recorded over 57,000 visits in 1973, including 19,000 complete and comprehensive visual examinations; and over 7000 vision training patients. "ICO's specialized clinic facilities and services include the finest optometric pathology amphitheater in the country, a low vision department which provides extensive services for the partially sighted, and a contact lens department continually involved in research ...The ICO Clinic is not only a valued community health resource, but had expanded its service to several affiliated clinics. At present time, our senior interns are assigned to 7 affiliated clinics, which we feel increases the clinical experience of the student intern through his participation in the delivery of optometric care under an interdisciplinary health facility, " explained Dr. Wal-

Baseball great Ernie Banks helped promote the 1977 ICO vision exhibition "Vision: Children's Gateway to the World" at the Chicago Museum of Science and Industry.

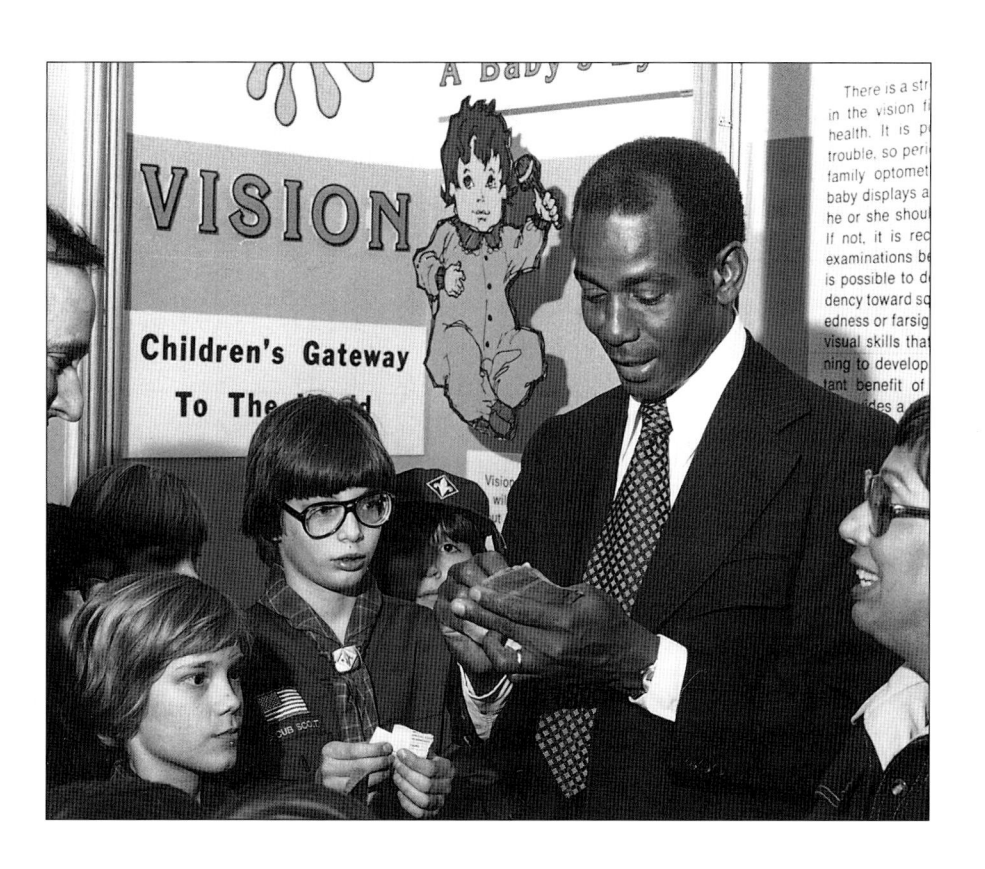

ter Yasko in his report to the *Journal of the Illinois Optometric Association.*[55]

During President Richard M. Nixon's administration, health maintenance organizations (HMOs) like California's Kaiser Plan offered the public a reasonably-priced, prepaid group health care service system which was launched with federal grants and loan guarantees. By 1971, there were at least 30 organizations in operation; and by 1978, the nation had 217 established groups.[56]

Optometry's role in the nation's health care system was reinforced once again by the federal Health Services and Centers Amendments of 1978 which described optometrists as the professionals "best suited by training and practice to deliver primary care vision services." Acknowledgment also came with increased coverage of optometric services by third-party insurance companies.[57]

The nation's educational system took advantage of the numerous federal grants offered between 1965 and 1980. Money was not only available for buildings and facilities, there were also additional funds for research. Like many health care institutions, ICO expanded its research department during this period.[58]

The contact lens department's faculty and students conducted hydrophilic and conventional contact lens research, in 1974, on volunteer ICO Eye Clinic patients under the faculty direction of Drs. John R. Roggenkamp, John Peterson, John Sharp, and Michael Politzer. (Roggenkamp had been appointed to be an FDA Researcher, in 1972, for the Ophthalmos Inc. Hydrolens which had not been approved but was under investigative exemption.) The department was also involved with clinical studies of other soft lenses, and a follow-up project on the application of soft lenses in astigmatic cases.[59]

ICO's clinical researchers investigated the visual, developmental and perceptual abilities of Down's syndrome

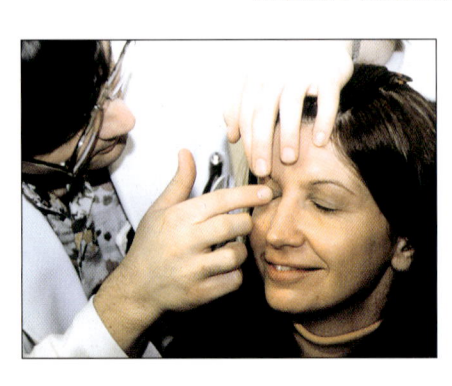

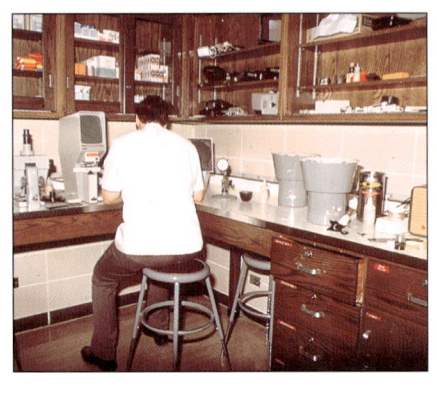

ICO students learned up-to-date contact lens fitting techniques in the school's clinic.

children; use of the Titmus Color Test for screening color deficiencies; the relationship between reading and short-term memory; and Silo response. Student researchers conducted additional studies on the use of tonometry in contact lens fitting. The pediatric clinic itself was redesigned in a modular formula that grouped general vision exam rooms for patients aged 3 to 12 with rooms for developmental vision evaluations and strabismus/amblyopia examinations along with a new clinic for the examination and treatment of vision problems in infants.[60]

The infant care clinic combined primary health care with optometric care. Opened in 1977, the clinic examined more than 100 patients in its first 6 months of operation, many of whom were referred to outside agencies specializing in infant problems.[61]

In the 1975 fall session, 150 new enrollees joined students in researching stereo blindness, and the basic physiological effects of the visual system. Studies were also conducted on the influence of contact lenses on corneal physiology; the differences between soft and hard contact lens use; the utility of contact lenses of various sizes; and sterility procedures in lens use. As the research committee chairman reported, "the research efforts at ICO

ICO students participating in the VOSH program gained valuable experience abroad while contributing to the vision health of disadvantaged people in Haiti and other areas.

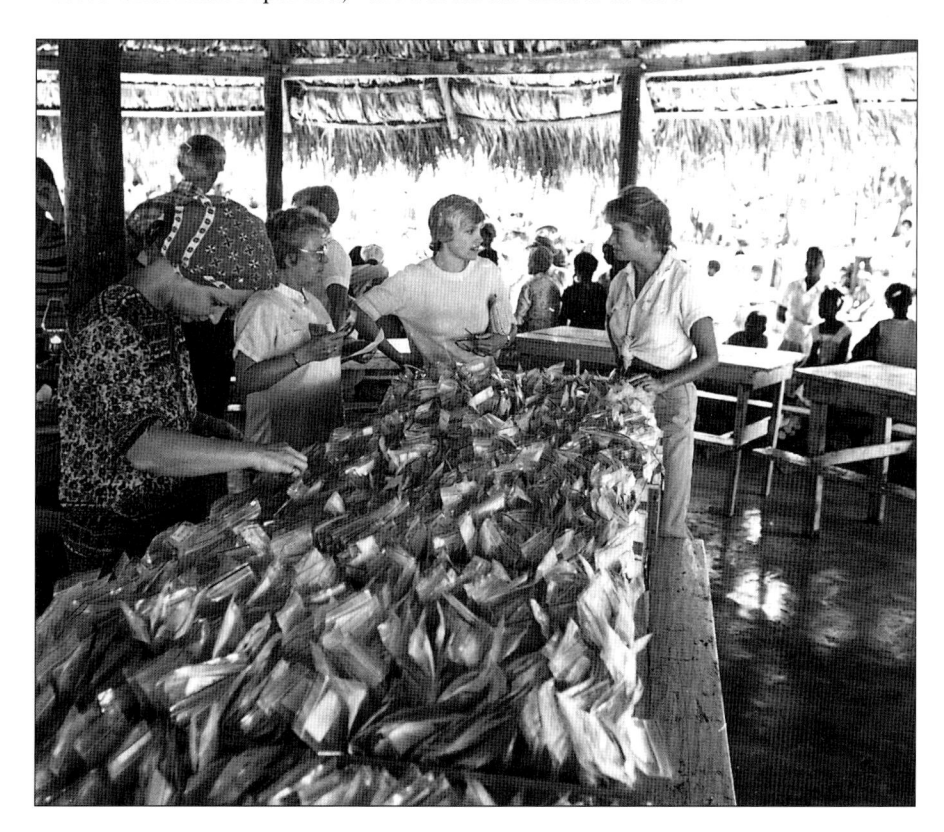

are improving in quality and quantity...not only faculty research, but also supervised student efforts. It is apparent that, given the necessary equipment and time, the college can and will develop a viable research program. This program will be of a very high quality."[62]

Outside of the school, a pair of CCO graduates were making contact lens history. Drs. Newton Wesley and George Jessen had met in the 1940s when Wesley was an instructor at Monroe College of Optometry. When Jessen graduated in 1945, the two formed a partnership called the Plastic Contact Lens Company. They became pioneers in many areas of hard contact lens design, manufacture, and fitting. During the 1970s, they renamed the company Wesley-Jessen, and commenced researching and developing soft contact lenses. Their work led to to the 1978 U.S. FDA approval of their hydrogel lens: a durable, highly-permeable, polymer-based lens. They also created a unique form of toric contact lens which turned out to be valuable in the treatment of some astigmatic cases.[63]

COMPUTERIZATION AND TRANSITION

IN 1975, the optometry and visual science departments acquired a $20,000 VER computer through a National Eye Institute grant. About the size of a home refrigerator, the computer had basic keyboard, a typewriter-style printer and no video terminal – though for its time it was state of the art. It was used primarily for research in the electrodiagnostic laboratory, but administrative staff shared time on it for bookkeeping, accounting and general business operations.[64]

Change had become a part of the school's ongoing process as it was still defining its identity in the educational system and growing with the profession. The late 1970s continued to highlight major shifts on every front, including the Board of Trustees and administrative personnel. Dr. Anthony Nizza became the first faculty member to head up the new ICO Eye Clinic Residency Program in 1978. The next year, Shane J. Conway was named ICO executive vice president; and Gregory W. Petty became dean of students. Another major transition occurred, in 1981, when Dr. Rosenbloom resigned his position as ICO's president and became the school's first Distinguished Professor of Optometry. By this time, ICO's foundations were firmly established and the school was ready to plan for the future.[65]

OPTOMETRY
IN AMERICA

102

Pediatric trial lens frames are often used to test for required lens strengths. Patients can try reading with various lenses at a variety of distances.

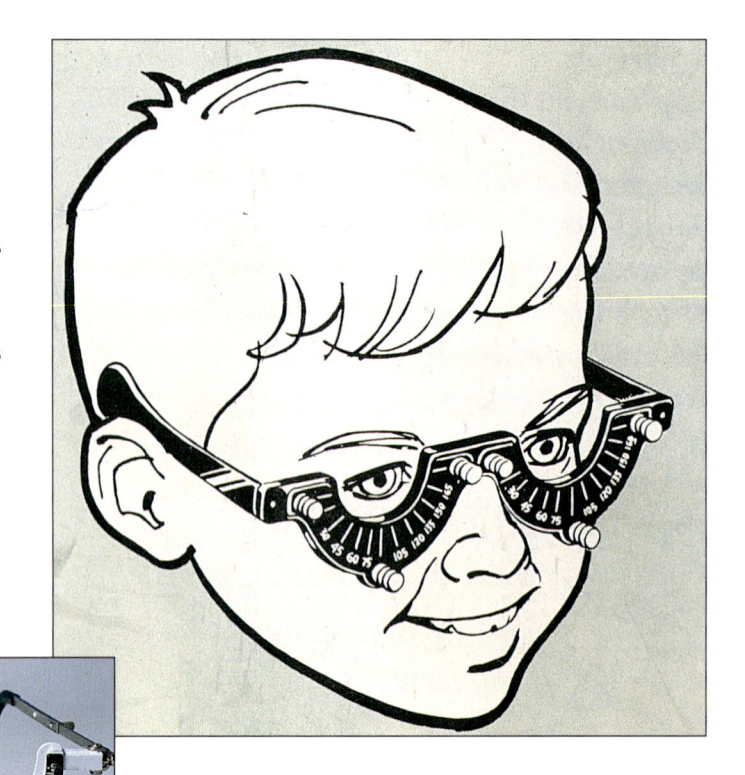

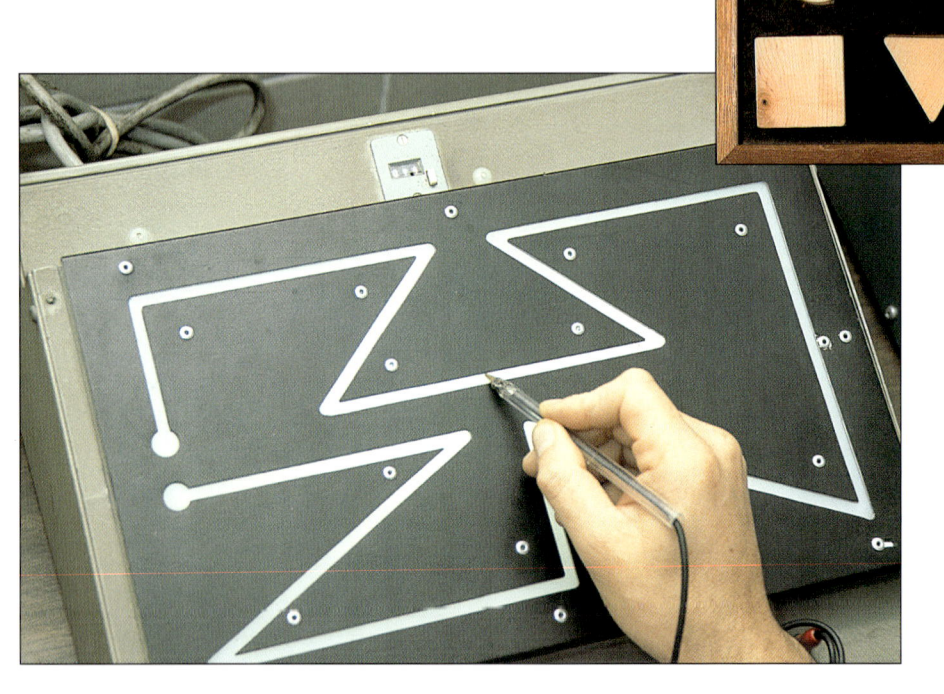

The Manas Maze (left) desgned by Dr. Leo Manas, and the craft form board (above) are valuable testing and vision training devices used in the pediatric clinic.

A NEWER WORLD
TO SEE

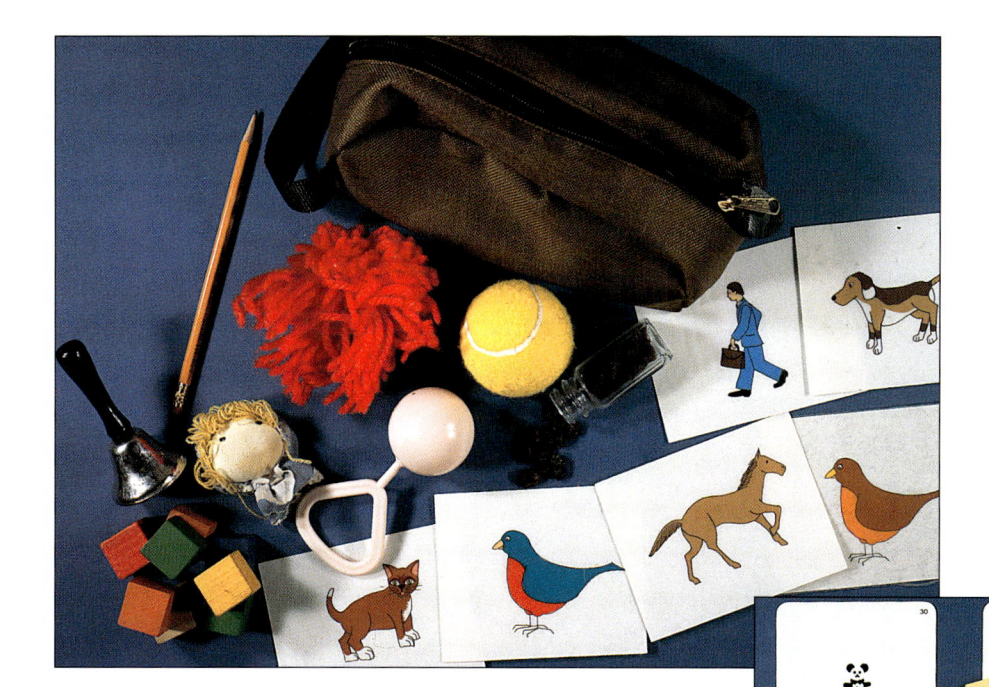

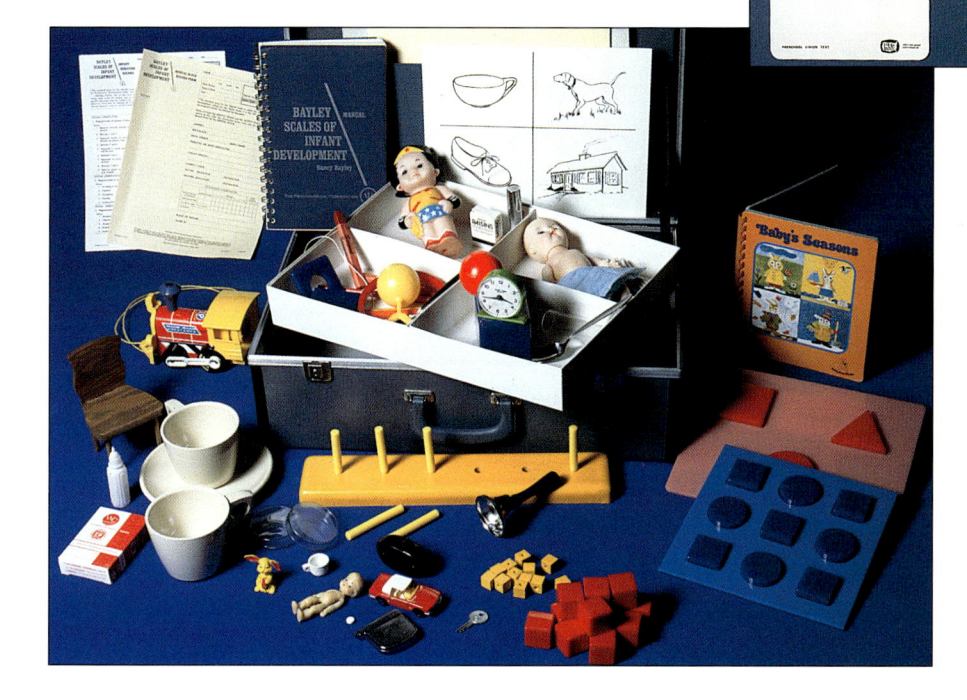

103

Developmental testing as it relates to vision takes many forms including The Denver Development test (top left); The Allen Cards (above); and the Bayley Scales (left) which are used for testing infant development.

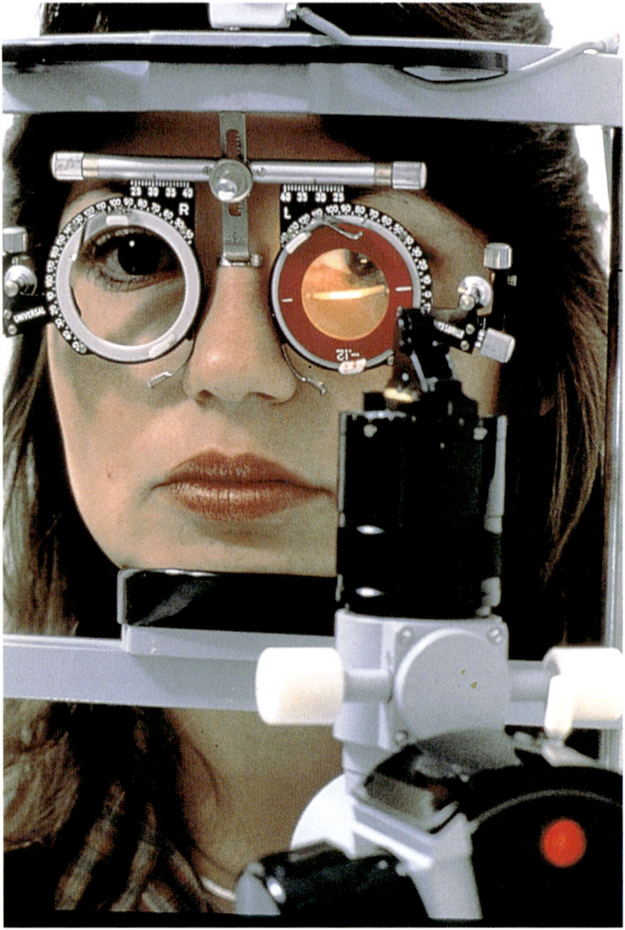
25 30 35 40
R
40 35 30 25
L
UNIVERSAL

CHAPTER 6

The FLAGSHIP

ILLINOIS COLLEGE OF OPTOMETRY'S
PRESENT AND ITS FUTURE

Looking toward its future as a leader in optometric education, ICO will continue to pioneer technological advances and set the pace for interdisciplinary primary care management.

EDUCATION SETS THE PACE

ILLINOIS COLLEGE OF OPTOMETRY'S President, Dr. Boyd B. Banwell, stated in a recent interview: "Most people think educational programs are secondary to optometric practice. They don't realize education sets the pace. You can go out and pass all the laws and legislation you want, but unless the colleges are prepared to handle it, you've done nothing."[1]

Approximately one-fourth of all American optometrists practicing today are graduates of ICO, NICO, or CCO. The 125-year history of ICO and its predecessors is hallmarked by impressive expansions of both its curriculum and campus, spurred by the equally meteoric growth of the optometric profession.

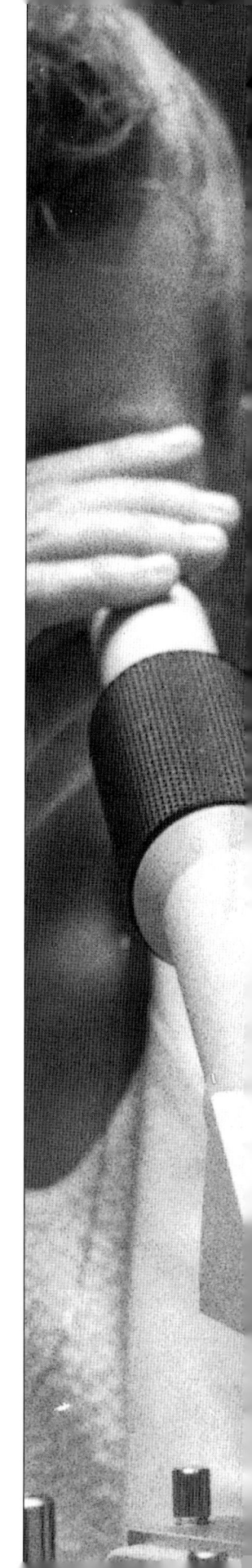

Today, ICO provides a 4-year, graduate-level professional program leading to a doctorate degree in optometry for the nation's largest optometric student body. Geared to handle approximately 600 students — nearly 4 times the size of the 1983 student body — ICO enrolled 590 students in its 1995-1996 session.

The AOA's Council on Optometric Education (COE) awarded ICO's doctorate program the maximum professional accreditation in 1988. The next year, the North Central Association of Schools and Colleges re-accredited ICO for their maximum period. In addition to its sterling institutional accreditation, ICO's post-doctoral primary care residency program has received the COE's maximum accreditation.

Students can choose from a wide variety of degree programs. ICO now awards a Bachelor of Science in Visual Science degree (B.S.V.S.), prior to the completion of the O.D. program, to students who complete one year's work in social studies, humanities, and foreign language in addition to their professional course work.[2]

The school has developed the nation's first combined O.D.-Ph.D. degree program, in association with Boston University's Division of Graduate Medical and Dental Sciences. The curriculum's clinical training takes place at ICO, while a non-clinical doctoral component in one of the basic medical sciences (neurobiology, biochemistry, pathology, etc.) is taken at Boston University. The first candidates for this degree were matriculated during the 1994-1995 academic year.[3]

ICO's educational program continues to combine classroom and laboratory instruction with intensive clinical training. Students spend their first 2 years focused on classroom and laboratory work in basic biomedical sciences. They also gain extensive clinical experience, which is carefully monitored and designed to acclimate them to the patient care environment. During the third year, students are integrated into direct patient care activities while continuing their classroom and laboratory training. The students' fourth year is devoted almost exclusively to clinic-oriented patient care activities, continued under the careful guidance of the clinic's teaching optometrists.

Daily clinical training throughout the program is designed to prepare students for their future roles as practicing optometrists. Under the direction of ICO's clinical education department chair, Dr. Dennis W. Siemsen, (who is also assistant dean for patient care) training takes place in interdisciplinary environments where students interact with a wide range of medical specialists — internists, neurologists, ophthalmologists — and infectious disease and pulmonary medicine subspecialists. (Dr. Siemsen also serves as the American Academy of Optometry's optometric education section chairman; and recently completed a term as the clinical skills education chairman of the National Board of Examiners in Optometry (NBEO).)

By the early 1990s, ICO's curriculum was recognized by the COE as one of the field's most comprehensive. Students are provided state-of-the-art medically-oriented courses presented by a faculty of nationally known medical, optometric and health care experts.

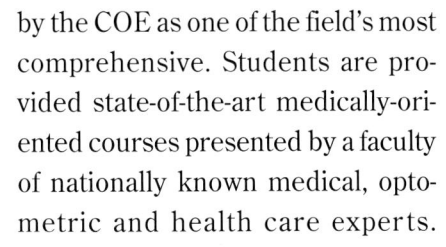

Practice opportunities for present and future optometrists have broadened considerably. Traditionally, optometrists worked in individual or small group practices. Now they are also finding their skills in demand in interdisciplinary health management teams, hospitals, and HMOs. These new opportunities have mandated that optometric educators continually expand and refine the curriculum. To meet that need, ICO has augmented its traditional faculty with many senior medical school educators and nationally recognized leaders in medical education and health care policy. Co-ordinated by Dr. Stanley Reiser, who is the Ross Professor of Humanities and Technology in Health Care at the University of Texas Health Sciences Center in Houston, Texas. These part-time faculty members provide more than a dozen fully integrated courses essential to both current and future optometric practice.

Many major metropolitan Chicago academic medical services and institutions have formed cooperative teaching relationships with ICO to enhance the courses. Among them

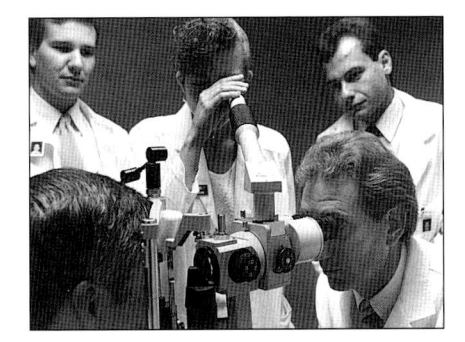

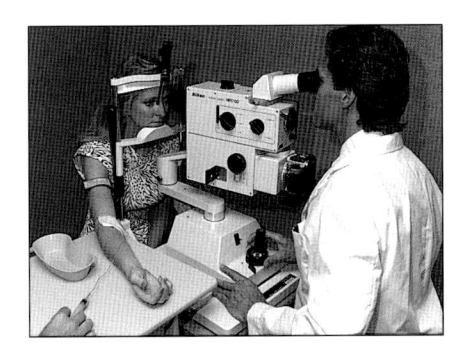

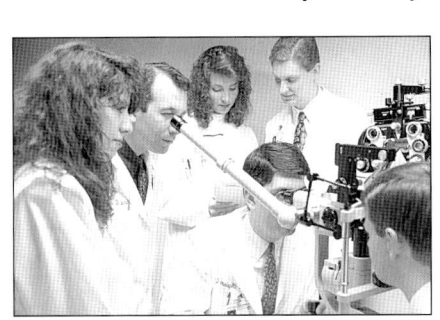

With the best teachers and equipment, students are thoroughly prepared for numerous opportunities opening up in their profession.

are: Rush Medical College's medicine, neurology, physiology and biochemistry departments and its infectious disease section; the University of Illinois (Chicago) College of Medicine's Department of Medical Education; and the University of Illinois' School of Public Health.

Another important measure of ICO's academic success can be found in ICO students' NBEO scores, which are required for licensing nationwide. Part I of NBEO encompasses basic sciences and was extensively revised three years ago to emphasize biomedical sciences. The revised NBEO Part I was administered for the first time in the spring of 1993. According to the official result data, ICO students averaged a score of 92 percent. The national average — including ICO students — was only 73 percent. ICO students have continued to score around 90 percent on first-take rounds of both the NBEO Part I and Part II since then. One hundred thirty-one ICO students took the NBEO Part III (Patient Care Examination) in 1995, which assesses graduates on their clinical skills. Those students scored an overall 94 percent — far above the national average.[4]

Applications have been increasing by about one-third annually in the past decade, and accepted enrollees far exceed the school's minimum requirements, making the student body the nation's most qualified. (Eighty-four percent of the school's 1993-1994 first-year students held pre-optometric bachelor's degrees prior to enrollment.) And in contrast to the high attrition rate of students just after the Second World War, ICO's present student attrition rate — due to withdrawal or academic deficiencies — is less than 5 percent annually.

A growing number of graduates from ICO and other colleges are seeking advanced and specialized clinical training beyond the 4-year program. The ICO postdoctoral program offers optometric graduates the opportunity to further enhance their clinical skills and to attain a certificate of completion. For those interested in optometric education as a career, the program also includes formal training from the health care education specialists of University of Illinois (Chicago) College of Medicine.

In addition to degree programs, ICO conducts postgraduate continuing education programs for practicing optometrists, covering many of the profession's latest

TPAs: therapeutic pharmaceutical agents such as topical anti-infectives, anti-allergics, anti-glaucomas, anti-inflammatories, over-the-counter topical formulas, non-narcotic oral analgesics, and mydriatics which are used in the treatment of certain eye conditions.

developments, like the application of diagnostic and therapeutic pharmaceutical agents (DPAs and TPAs).

In 1988, legislation was enacted nationwide authorizing optometrists to use DPAs in their examination procedures. With this and other significant developments in mind, American optometric educators must not only address traditional treatment of vision problems but also train students in the diagnosis of eye diseases and the application of general and ocular pharmacology as part of a comprehensive treatment program.

During 1993, ICO sponsored and conducted more than a dozen courses (ranging in length from half day seminars to 120-hour/14-day programs) attended by over 600 participants. The school's faculty are also frequently featured lecturers at major continuing education programs sponsored by organizations like the American Academy of Optometry (ICO had 30 presenters at the Academy's 1995 New Orleans meeting) and various state optometric associations.

ICO's students come from all over continental North America and overseas, including a 19 percent minority student population. The student body is almost equally composed of male and female students. According to the AOA there are currently 28,900 full-time American practitioners of whom 23 percent are female. In view of the enrollment ratios, the association speculates that by the turn of the century, this figure will rise to 30 percent.[5]

A member of the Illinois State Board of Examiners and a private practitioner with strong international health care experience, Dr. Millicent Knight, is a prime example of the profession's future. As an IEI pediatric patient, Dr. Knight had early contact with both the profession and the school. She recalled in an interview, "Since I was 6 years old, I always felt a genuine concern from the clinicians here, and I knew I wanted to go into the health field. I remember the clinician who fit my first pair of contact lenses at age seventeen. Years later, he remembered me, too. I had asked so many questions about optometry, he took me down to the Admissions Office."[6]

Prior to her 1987 graduation from ICO, Dr. Knight participated in the school's VOSH program, going on humanitarian missions to Columbia, Guatemala, and Costa Rica. She gained further experience before entering into

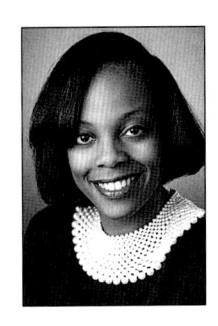

Once an IEI patient, Dr. Millicent Knight, was so inspired by the care she received at the clinic, she made the decision to become an optometrist when she grew older.

private practice by working in an interdisciplinary setting at a Chicago hospital-based eye center and participating in a 1991 Surgical Eye Expeditions project in Brazil that provided both pre- and post-operative care for poverty-stricken patients. As one of 45 national participants in the 3-year W.K. Kellogg Foundation National Fellowship Program (designed to help qualified professionals explore new interdisciplinary experiences on both national and international levels), Dr. Knight has continued to develop and broaden her knowledge not only of her chosen profession, but of its role in health care.[7]

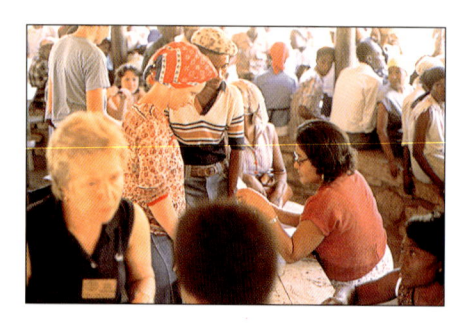

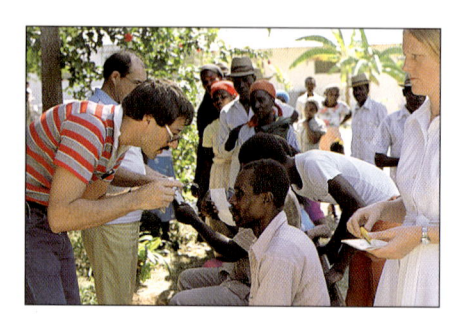

ICO students participating in VOSH have gained experience in such globally divergent areas as U.S. Indian reservea, Caribbean and Latin American nations, bringing aid to people who might never receive vision care otherwise.

Staffing these many programs is a faculty of 108 teachers who collectively hold an equal number of doctorates (O.D.s, M.D.s, and Ph.D.s). Sixty are full-time faculty members, including 13 who exclusively teach and supervise students and clinical residents in the school's off-campus affiliated programs. Twenty-eight of the 48 part-time faculty exclusively participate in the IEI's clinical education programs; 20 are regular course lecturers in subjects like the biomedical sciences, and many are senior faculty at area medical schools. As ICO's vice president of academic affairs and dean Dr. David A. Greenberg remarked, "the college is very proud of the role that its faculty has played in the recent evolution of our profession. ICO faculty have maintained leadership positions in numerous key optometric organizations over the past decade, including the NBEO, the American Academy of Optometry, COVD, and many more. In addition, our faculty's rate of publication has been extraordinary. Their articles regularly appear in all the major optometric journals and ophthalmic texts — many of which also utilize ICO faculty in editorial roles."[8]

ICO's faculty is actively involved in advancing the profession's body of knowledge. One example is Dr. Stuart Richer, a part-time faculty member who is a principal investigator in the Macular Degeneration Study Group. The team has been conducting a 3-year pilot study of the relationship between atrophic ARMD and nutrition. Like glaucoma, atrophic ARMD is largely undetectable in its early stages. This chronic, vision degenerating disease affects many older people whose lifetime dietary seem to be high in fats and lacking in critical nutrients. The study demonstrated that there is reason to believe dietary antioxidants and reduced fat intake may have some preventive effect during the disease's early stages.

Breaking away the traditional system of tenure followed by most American colleges and universities, ICO adopted a renewable-contract tenure system in 1982. The program secures associate professors for 4 academic years, and full professors for 6 academic years. This program allows the school to review and evaluate its faculty's ability to match the educational program's needs and to keep pace with advances in the profession. The COE noted "it is clear that the faculty is empowered and assumes significant responsibility in all faculty governance areas, …There is considerable vitality in these areas with committees actively functioning and contributing to the growth of the institution. In summary, the governing process is continuous, dynamic and effective. It encourages and supports faculty ownership of the academic process."

THE MAYO CLINIC IN EYE CARE

"IN THE BEGINNING," Dr. Banwell stated in a recent interview, "I told the board that we will make this the Mayo Clinic of eye care in the Midwest." In his 13 years in office, he has worked unceasingly toward that primary goal.[9] (Banwell was inaugurated in 1983, with former President Gerald R. Ford as the keynote speaker.[10])

At age 14, Banwell never would have guessed what the future had in store for him. He was running a fishing boat on Burt Lake in Michigan for his father's charter company. He was

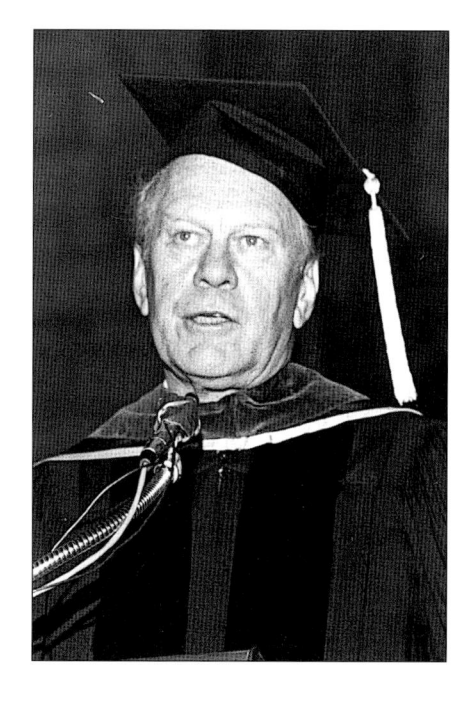

The speaker for Dr. Banwell's inauguration was former U.S. President Gerald R. Ford, whose brother is an optometrist.

the youngest person ever to earn a charter license on the Great Lakes. But he knew the value of good vision early in life. He had a vision problem as a child; an oculist prescribed glasses and told him he had a "bad eye." When Banwell's interest turned to science, he chose optometry as his future profession. After serving in the Second World War, and earning a bachelor of science degree at Wayne State University, Banwell enrolled at NICO. He graduated in 1954 and established a successful private practice in Williamston, Michigan, near Lansing. During his 3 decades in the profession, Banwell also became a very active member of the AOA and the Michigan Optometry Association. (He was elected president of MOA.) Hoping to make a lasting impact on the quality and availability of vision care, he became an optometric lobbyist for the establishment of the Michigan Medicaid Program and Ferris State University in the late 1960s.[11]

Dr. Banwell became concerned about his alma mater (now ICO) when the school became heavily involved in a federally-funded expansion program. He was elected to ICO's board in 1969 and served for 6 years as finance committee chairman. He was then elected board chairman in 1974. During that time, he led ICO's efforts to acquire additional land for the campus' future expansion while striving to minimize the school's debt load. He served as interim president before he was appointed ICO president in January 1982.[12]

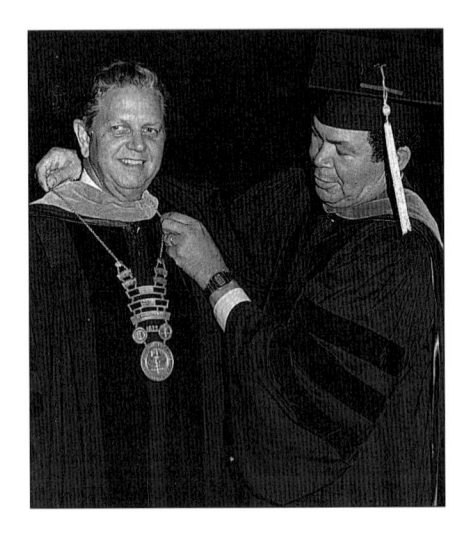

Past chairman of the Board of Trustees Dr. Joseph L. Henry presented Dr. Banwell with the seal of the President.

Once in office, he instituted a 10-year plan to improve the school's financial stability; update and expand its equipment and facilities; and reorganize its academic program. His overriding goal was the establishment of ICO as an educational leader well into the next century. By the early 1990s, those goals were being fully realized and Dr. Banwell was well on his way to planning the next decade of purposeful, progressive expansion.[13]

In 1995, a couple of landmark legislative decisions affected the academic needs of incoming students. Illinois Senate Bill 185, allowing certified Illinois optometrists to utilize TPAs in their practices was signed into law. Illinois

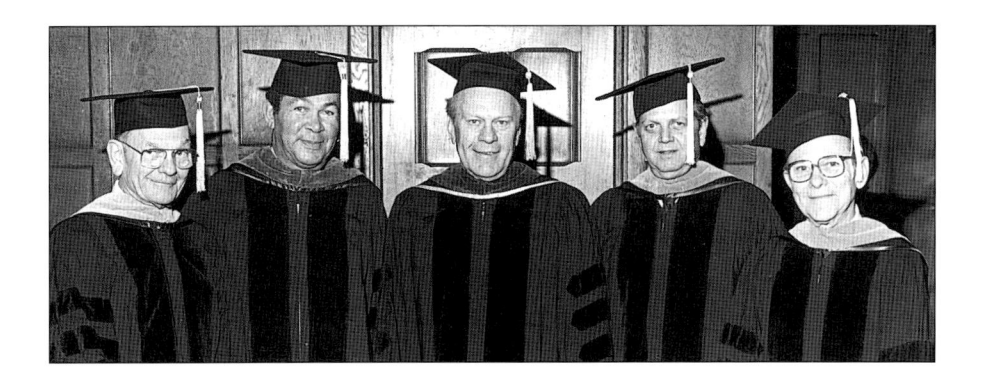

(From left to right) Drs. C.K. Hill, Joseph L. Henry, Boyd B. Banwell, and Dr. Frederick Kushner posed with President Gerald R. Ford (center) at Banwell's inauguration.

became the forty-fifth state to establish TPA legislation. Optometric legislation in the 1980s allowed certified optometrists to use DPAs in patient examinations. But under this new law, Illinois optometrists were given authority to treat "any ocular abnormality, disease, or visual or muscular anomaly of the human eye or visual system;" provide any non-surgical ophthalmic emergency care; and remove superficial foreign bodies from patients' eyes and surrounding tissues.[14]

According to Banwell: "TPA rights for optometrists are in the best interest of Illinois citizens. This law will allow for greater patient accessibility to treatment, particularly for residents living in rural areas where there are fewer ophthalmologists. We have been teaching the necessary courses to prepare our graduating optometrists for the day this bill would be passed." Banwell championed the bill's legislation for nearly a decade, and had already established an academic program to cover not only detection and treatment of ocular disease, but participation in the management of systemic disorders. Consequently, ICO graduates, whether practicing in states that had enacted similar legislation early on or not, were entering the field fully qualified.[15]

The second landmark legislative action to take place that year was the passage of an amendment to the Illinois Optometric Practice Act. As its most outspoken proponent, Banwell explained, "With this ammendment's passage we became an independent profession. We had legislation passed called 'as taught' legislation. We don't have to go back to the legislature. If something develops, if we develop something, we go through a procedure — the rules committee, the state board of examiners, the department of licensing. We can then practice what is taught." Earli-

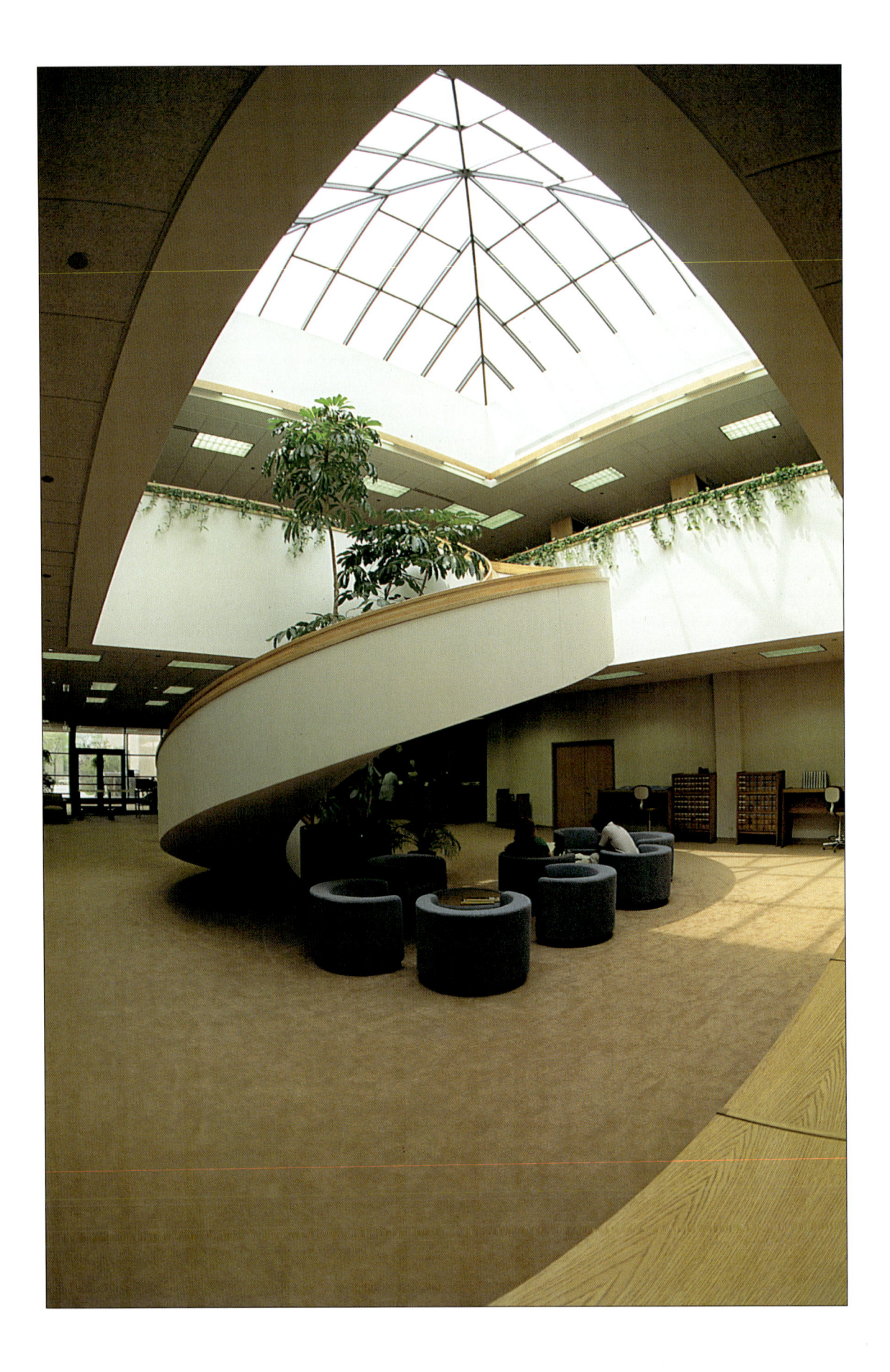

er, when DPAs were permitted in Illinois, a technical review board — consisting of pharmacists, 2 optometrists, and 2 ophthalmologists — was established to govern optometric practice. "Even though we taught a full complement of eye care right on through treatment, they had governing power," Banwell remembered. "So we eliminated that technical review board in this legislation. …We're off and running and setting the pace for the optometric profession."[16]

But Banwell's foresight is tempered by his firm belief in an essential foundation: "There's a lot of things we have to look at. But I always want to see us interested in optometry as it grew up: in the interest of patient care — to make it more convenient for patients to get proper eye care. Use the subspecialties — retinal surgery and treatment of the exotic diseases — those need to be done by specialists because that's all they do. When you're on ice that thin, you need the best you can get and everybody can't do everything."[17]

To create an academic program able to prepare future students to provide high-quality care in specialized fields as well as traditional settings, Dr. Banwell appointed Dr. David A. Greenberg, a 1974 New England College of Optometry graduate, as ICO's vice president for academic affairs and dean in 1984. He had joined the school earlier that same year as its executive director for institutional planning.[18]

Since he assumed the office of dean, Greenberg has created a strong educational base that integrates community involvement, multidisciplinary cooperation, and fosters an atmosphere in which students can reach a level of practical independence prior to their graduation. As the

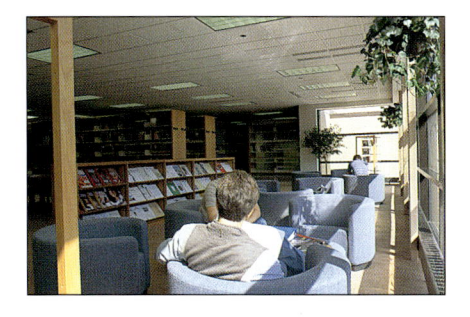

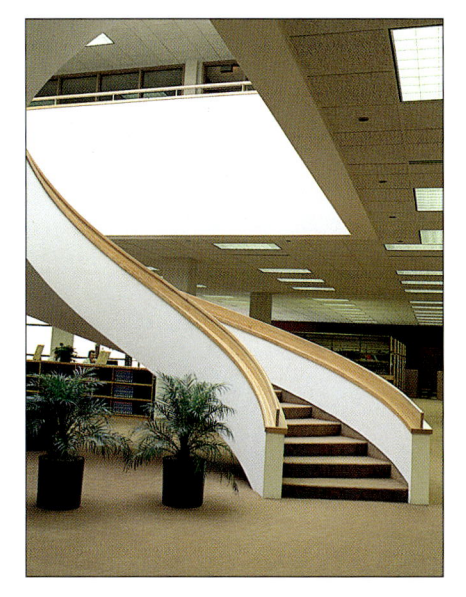

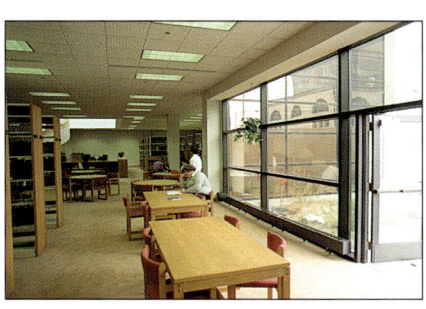

The ICO library, complete with a video library and computer workstations for students and faculty, was completed in 1985.

COE stated: "The curriculum has been changed and continually refined to be concordant with the cutting edge of the knowledge base and clinical training that prepares graduates to practice at the full scope of optometry."[19]

ICO's board of trustees includes immediate past chairman Dr. Joseph B. Ebbeson, treasurer Benjamin S. Wolfe, Dr. Ward R. Ransdell, Dr. Albert H. Rodriguez, Jr., Dr. Howard J. Woolf, Nancy Philip, and alumni trustee Dr. James Butler. Also within its membership are representatives of ICO's long history and nationally prominent figures who support the breakthrough programs that have been implemented and the future plans that will bring ICO into the next century. Former board chairman Dr. W. Judd Chapman is also an AOA past president and former chairman of the AOA's pubic information service. Secretary and past chairman Dr. C.K. Hill is a past-president of the ICO Alumni Council. Assistant treasurer and past chairman Dr. Frederick R. Kushner chaired the AOA's practice management committee. Dr. Joseph L. Henry, dean of Howard University School of Dentistry, was one of the first African-American dentists to receive a doctorate in any field. And present chairman Dr. John E. Brandt is past chairman of the Florida Optometric Association's Committee on Continuing Education.[20]

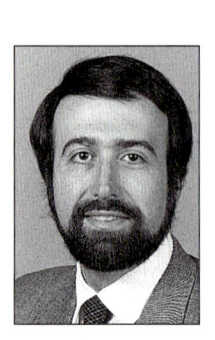

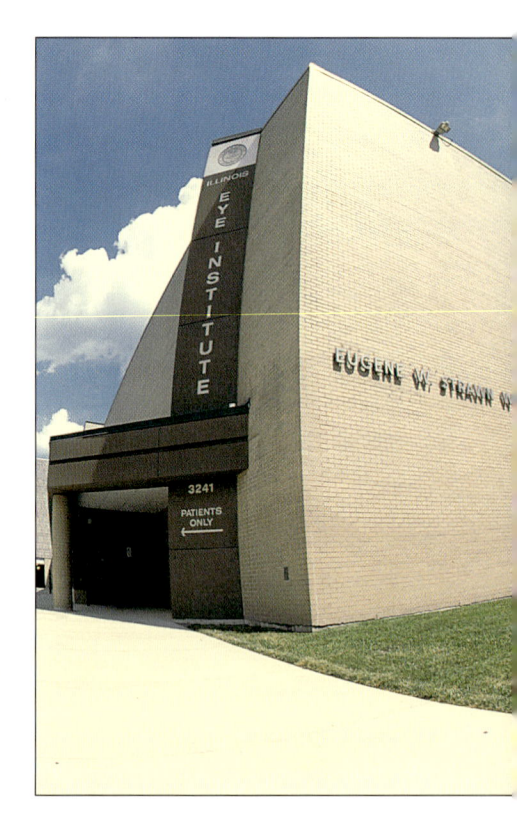

Dr. David A. Greenberg became vice-president for academic affairs and dean in 1984.

The new Illinois Eye Institute building houses a state-of-the-art facility for treating vision patients.

TO PROVIDE THE BEST

ILLINOIS EYE INSTITUTE handles more than 65,000 scheduled patient visits annually on campus and an additional 25,000 patients at IEI's full-time affiliated clinics. IEI's Executive Director Barbara Hamu served as administrator of Mt. Sinai Hospital Medical Center's Sinai Medical Group, Ltd., and its multi-specialty group operations before joining ICO. Along with staff and faculty guidance, students experience diverse, comprehensive clinical work that accurately reflects as broad a spectrum of cases as they could ever be faced with in professional practice. IEI's patients range from infants through senior citizens with a wide variety of ocular pathologies. Students also examine a large number of special-needs patients who utilize IEI's specialty services.[21]

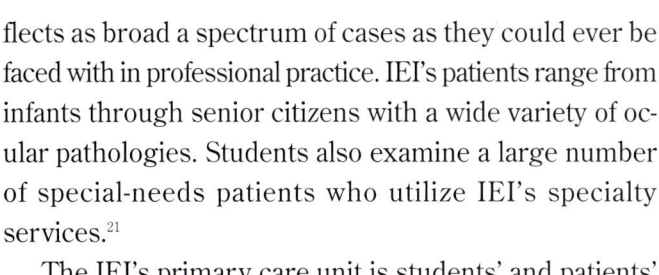

The IEI's primary care unit is students' and patients' entry to the clinical system. Students practice the basic necessary optometric screening techniques and procedures by examining patients.

In addition to serving patients with advanced contact lens care, IEI's cornea and contact lens service provides a wide variety of special services for patients requiring cosmetic masking or corneal and anterior segment eye disease treatment.

It is estimated that approximately 1 in 4 American children has an eye disorder. If not corrected by age 6, many of these disorders can result in vision impairment with lifelong consequences. Pediatric eye care emphasizes early assessment and intervention to facilitate and maximize a child's ability to develop normal vision. ICO students learn the application of specialized knowledge and methodologies in pediatric care for infants, preschoolers and grade school children in IEI's binocular vision/pediatric care service. Specialized instrumentation is used to detect and treat vision disorders — like myopia, strabismus, and amblyopia. When necessary, vision training is also provided for patients.

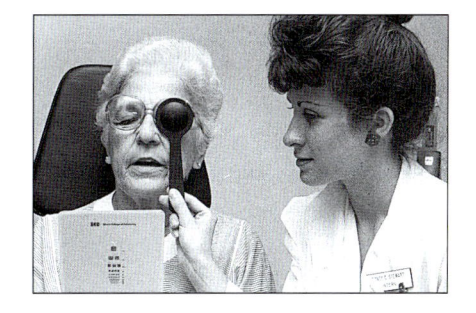

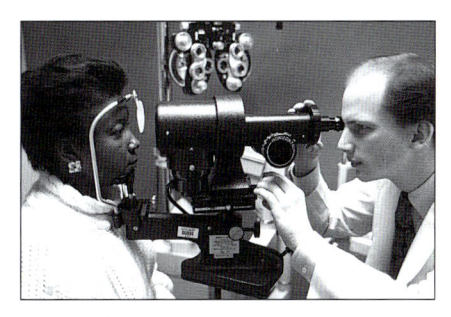

Information on the functional visual abilities of developmentally disabled children is gathered and disseminated. In consultation with speech and language specialists, this assessment is used to determine the optimal communication technology for these challenged children.

Fragile X syndrome — one of the most commonly inherited forms of mental retardation next to Down syndrome — affects 1 in 1000 men and 1 in 2000 women. Identified in 1991, this genetic disorder (which was orig-

THE FLAGSHIP

In the clinic, students work with as broad a range of patients as they would ever encounter in their professional careers.

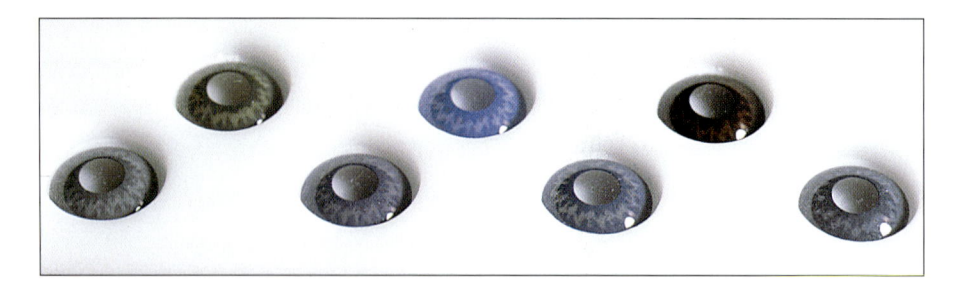

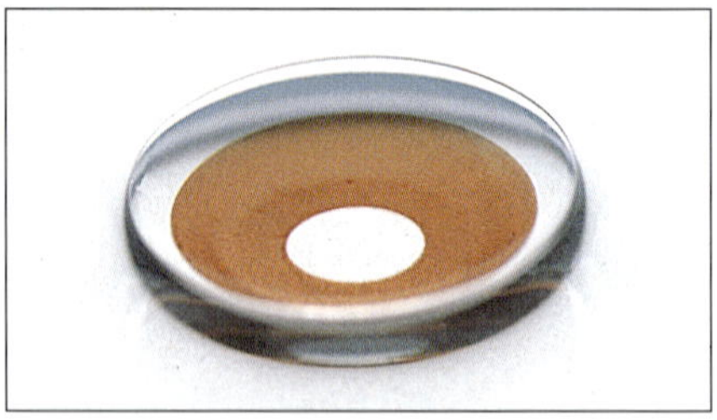

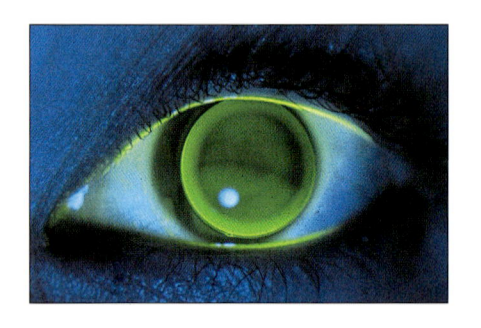

inally called Martin Bell syndrome) has among its many mild to severe physical traits vision malfunctions that contribute to other psychological, behavioral, and developmental disabilities. In conjunction with Rush Presbyterian-St. Luke's Medical Center's Fragile X Clinic, IEI's binocular vision/pediatric care service provides specialized screening and support services including evaluation and treatment. Because of the disease's interdisciplinary nature, the program is co-managed by IEI faculty in conjunction with other consulting medical professionals.[22]

It is estimated that as many as 15 million Americans — typically seniors — have permanent visual impairments caused by disease that cannot be corrected with eyeglasses or contact lenses. These functional impairments can often be significantly reduced by the application of carefully-prescribed, specialized devices such as telescopes and closed-circuit televisions. IEI's Center for Advanced Ophthalmic Care is also equipped for patient examinations where services require IEI consultants specializing in vitreoretinal or other ophthalmic surgery.

Ultrasonography and electrodiagnostic testing, utilizing highly-sophisticated instrumentation to obtain indirect electronic measures of visual function, are provided by the center. These are particularly useful for screening infants and older patients with communication difficulties which may preclude normal examination methods. In addition to their regularly scheduled hours, the center has also maintained a 24-hour walk-in emergency vision care service with an ocular emergency suite since 1991. It is

Advances continue to be made in both corrective and cosmetic contact lenses.

One of the most rewarding of an optometrist's duties, pediatric care can impact a child's entire life, opening new horizons.

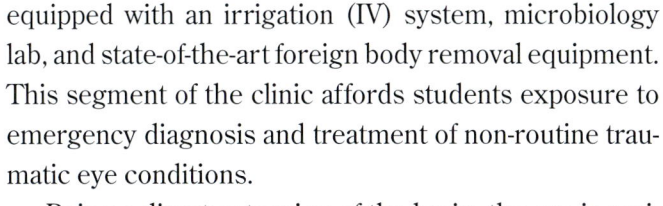

equipped with an irrigation (IV) system, microbiology lab, and state-of-the-art foreign body removal equipment. This segment of the clinic affords students exposure to emergency diagnosis and treatment of non-routine traumatic eye conditions.

Being a direct extension of the brain, the eye is easily affected by common neurologic diseases such as multiple sclerosis. Impaired vision is the first symptom to become evident in approximately 25 percent of these cases. Neuro-ophthalmic evaluation by ICO optometrists provides critical early diagnosis leading to prompt intervention by the clinic's consulting neurologists.

Many of IEI's impoverished, inner city patients go for years without a medical check-up. But because eye trouble is difficult to ignore, they arrive at the clinic. In addition to multiple sclerosis, students are trained to spot diabetes, high blood pressure, along with a host of other diseases, and often save patients' lives by referring them to hospitals in time for medical attention.

In a survey conducted by the Easter Seal Society of Metropolitan Chicago, it was discovered that nearly 90 percent of community-based rehabilitation center patients who needed vision care had never received it. Underwritten by the United Way, the Amoco Foundation, and the Washington Square Health Foundation, IEI stepped in to serve these developmentally disabled patients as part of the Illinois Eye Institute-Easter Seals Eye Care Program since 1991, further broadening students' experience in diagnosing and managing special care patients.[23]

Maximum athletic performance is highly dependent upon good vision,

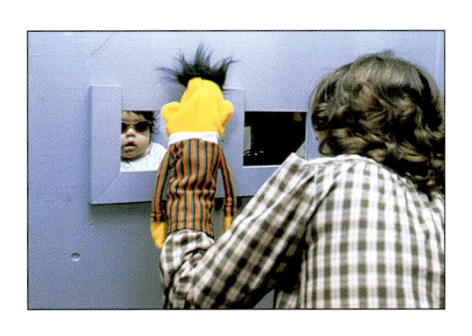

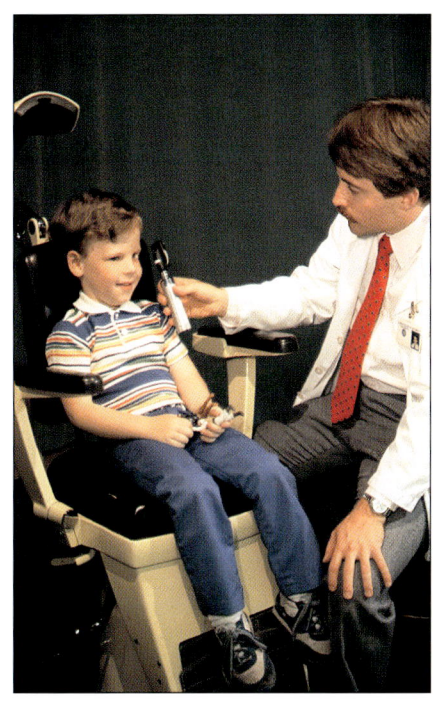

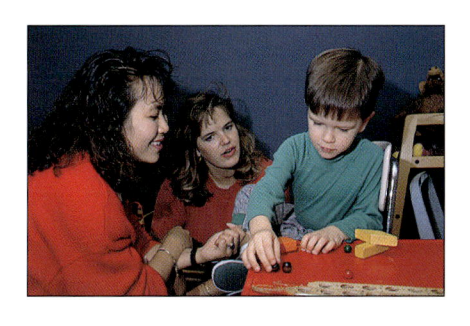

THE FLAGSHIP

119

yet 12 percent of the nation's amateur and professional athletes have insufficient visual acuity and many others are generally risking severe eye injury (90 percent of these injuries are preventable). The sports vision service has been screening and educating athletes since 1983. The examination involves 36 task related tests used to determine the existence and nature of any visual deficiency.[24]

Dedicated to helping both amateur and professional athletes attain their true potential, the Sports Vision Service has screened the members of the Chicago White Sox, the Montreal Expos, the Chicago Bulls, and varsity teams from De Paul University, University of Illinois (Chicago), Illinois Institute of Technology, Loyola University, the College of Du Page, and Illinois Benedictine. Faculty members like Dr. Stephen Beckerman, the head of Sports Vision Service, have also performed vision assessments on U.S. Olympic and Academy of Golf athletes.[25]

In an interview, Dr. Banwell added that sports vision is most valuable "if you introduce it into the lower grades, when kids are participating in Little League baseball and other youth sports. Then, as they correct, as they develop, they'll be better athletes. After all, every child deserves the chance to excel." ICO is also conducting public education campaigns to encourage parents and schools to have children's vision screened in schools. Numerous public and private schools (including the University of Chicago Laboratory School) are already participating in this outreach program.[26]

The IEI also houses a weekday family practice medical service staffed by Rush Presbyterian-St. Luke's Medical Center. In addition to the on-campus IEI, the school conducts full-time instructional clinic programs staffed by ICO faculty optometrists at 11 affiliated sites, including 9 teaching hospitals. Affiliations with organizations like the Maryville Academy for Youth (a Northern Illinois medical and residential facility caring for over 10,000 abused, abandoned, and neglected children) provide fourth-year students with additional experience and bring health care to those in

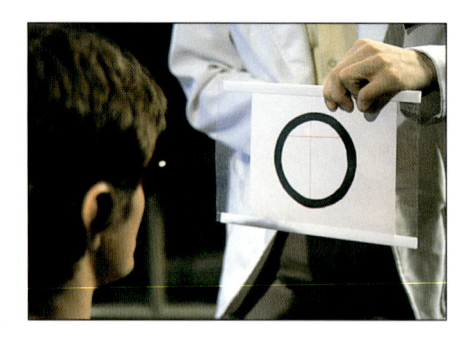

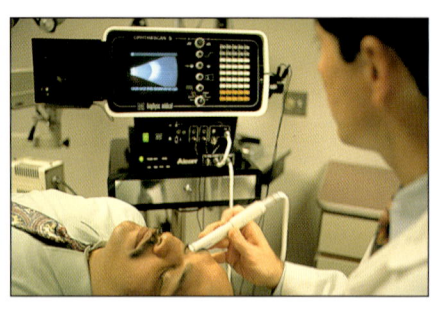

Advances in low vision care and vision training have brought sight to many people who might never have had a chance to live full and rewarding lives in the past.

THE FLAGSHIP

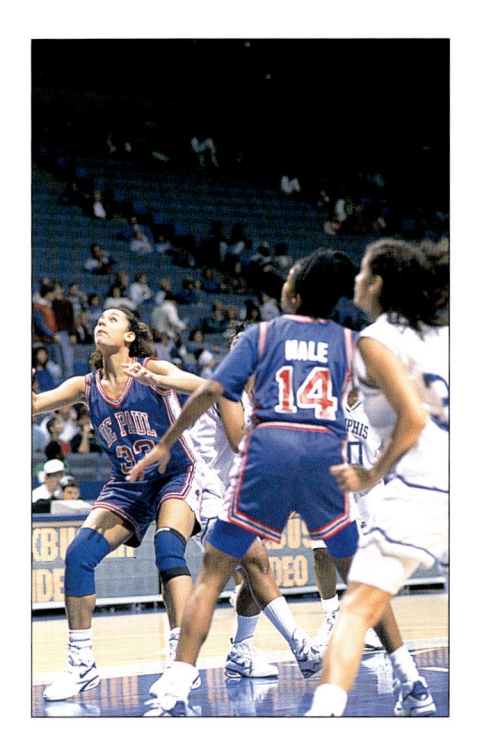

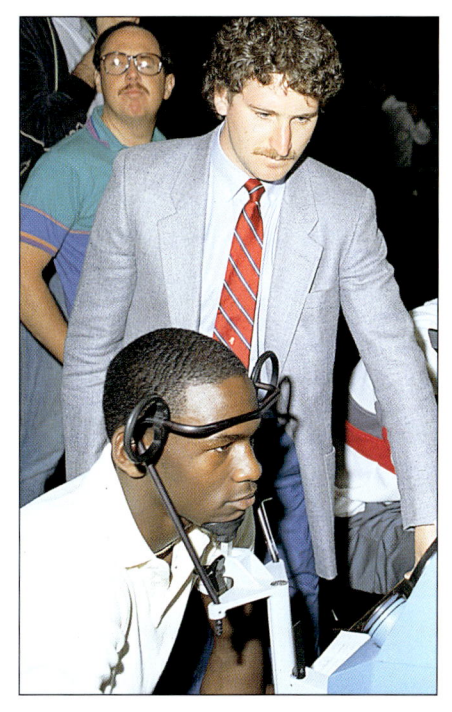

121

IEI clinicians working in the sports vision program tested Chicago Bull's player Michael Jordan. Needless to say his visual acuity is near perfect, but the program helps other professional and aspiring young athletes enhance their game by improving their vision.

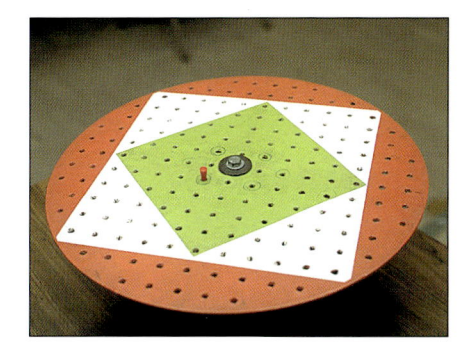

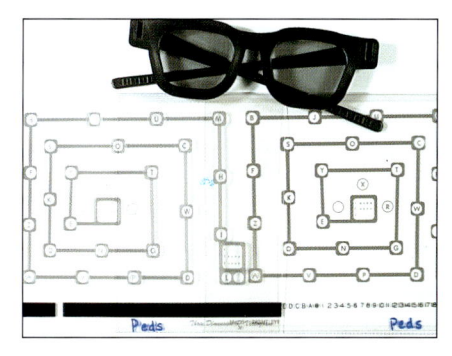

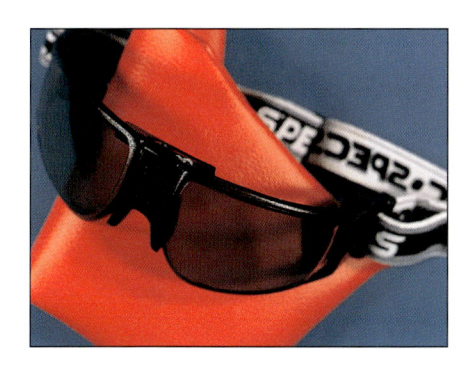

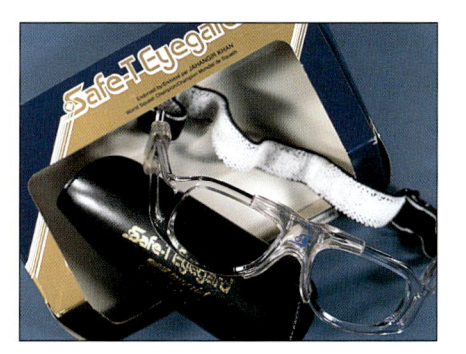

OPTOMETRY
IN AMERICA

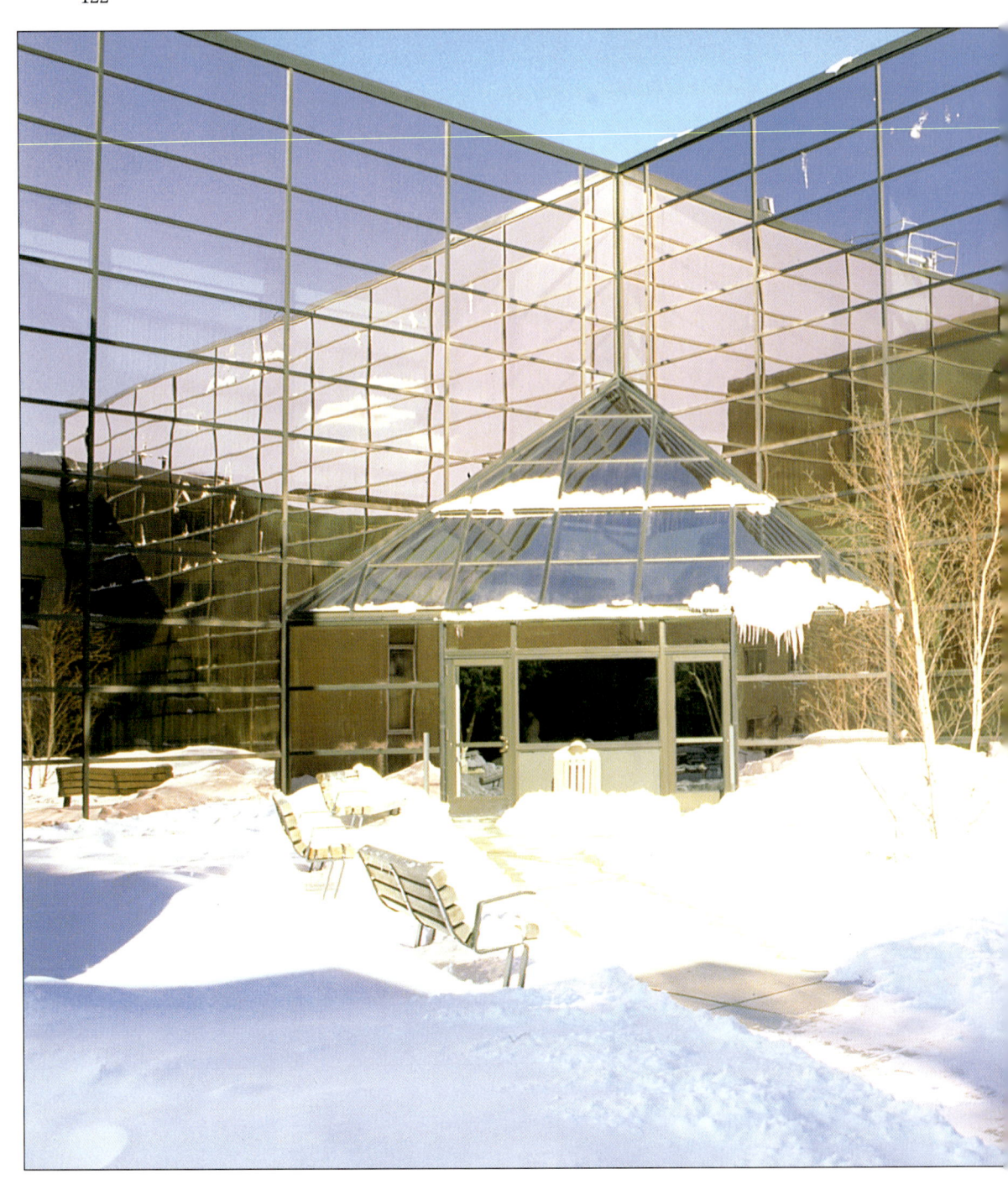

122

THE FLAGSHIP

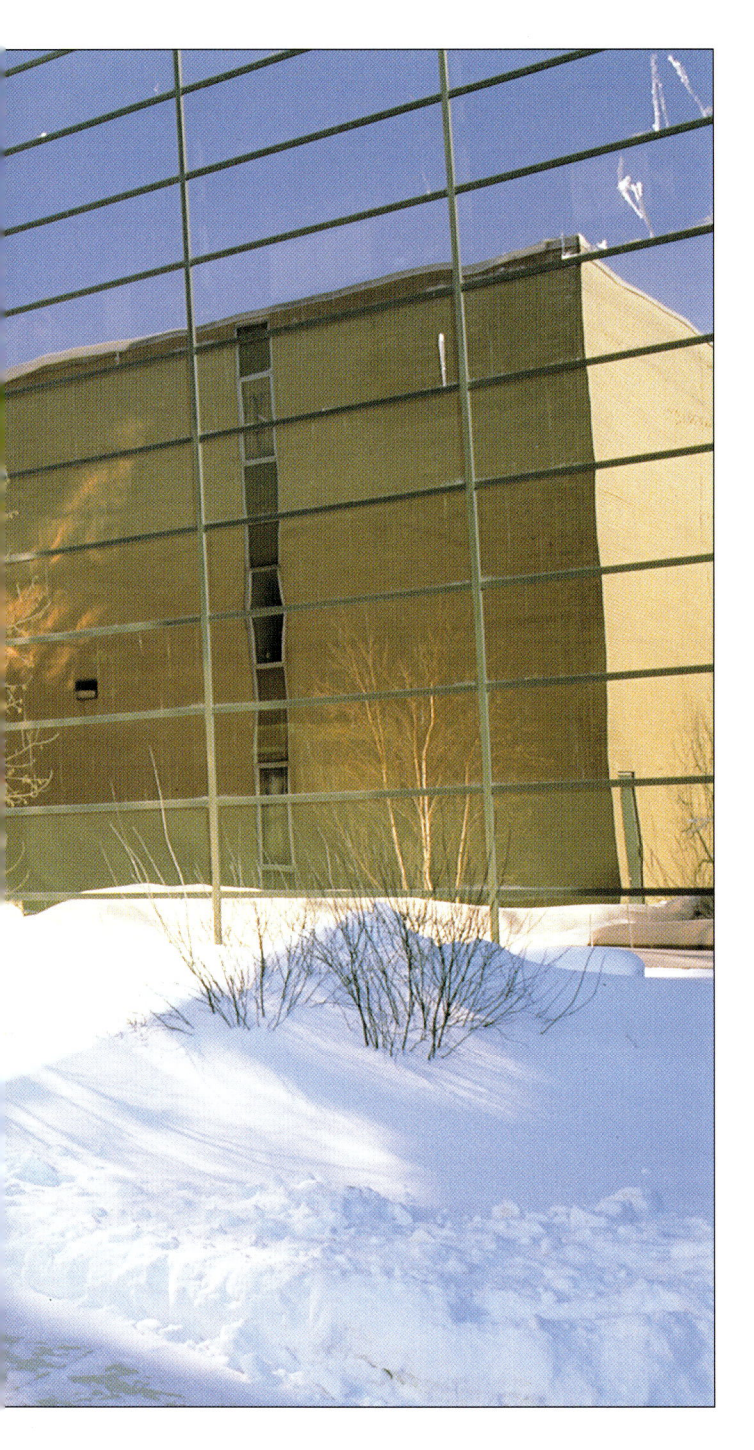

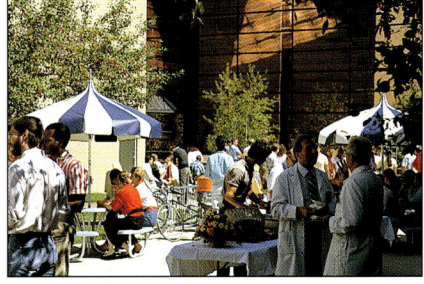

123

The school's courtyard is a popular gathering spot, and, in warm weather, it is frequently used for on-campus get-togethers.

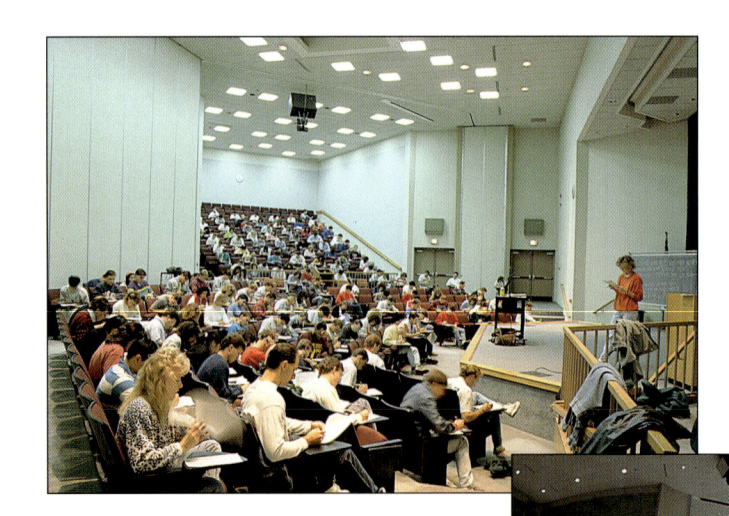

need. IEI conducts public vision and health screenings at public elementary school and Chicago Housing Authority "wellness fairs." Students also provide much-needed services at national off-campus sites like the Veterans Administration Medical Centers in Cleveland, Ohio and Huntington, West Virginia.

ICO's lecture center features A/V capabilities and the flexibility to convert into four smaller rooms when required.

ROOM TO GROW

IN THE SPRING OF 1982, construction commenced on a 50,000-square-foot building addition which included additional library space, a new auditorium, a lecture center, an outdoor study courtyard, administrative offices, a multi-story enclosed parking garage, a gymnasium/exercise facility, and a major clinic renovation. When it was completed in 1985, ICO's facilities expanded to approximately 213,000 square feet, forming a unified educational and patient care complex. The design received an excellence in architecture award in 1988 from The Northeast Illinois Chapter of the American Institute of Architects.

The new lecture center readily converts from 4 A/V equipped 160-seat independent modular lecture halls into a single 700-seat amphitheater. The learning resource center also contains a student computer center (with national on-line research capability), a fully-equipped, in-house television and video production studio, student A/V center, photographic, and desk-top publishing services which are all

THE FLAGSHIP

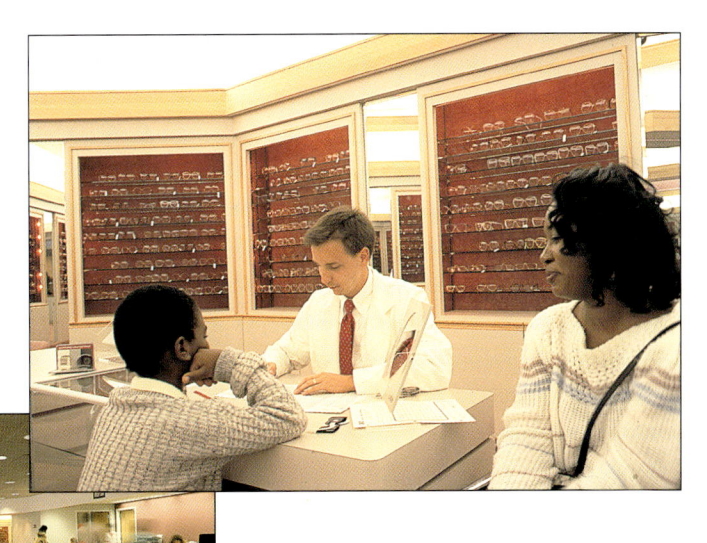

The clinic's facilities include a complete eyewear dispensary located next to the patient waiting area.

used to enhance the quality of teaching materials and facilitate student research.

IEI has been expanded to approximately 40,000 square-feet containing 92 examining rooms, clinical amphitheater, patient registration and reception areas, and a dispensing area.

In 1988, the entire ground floor of the Strawn Wing was completed and dedicated by Illinois Governor James Thompson. There are plans to incorporate the nearby Vandercook College of Music building into ICO's facilities in the near future.

Additional 1993 renovations included 14 additional faculty offices, a faculty lounge, an expanded student financial aid area; a new student services area, new IEI patient care areas including: 2 more primary care suites (each consisting of 8 examination rooms and a consultation room), and a sports vision area.

Dr. Banwell explained: "It's a matter of planning: orchestrating the logistics of putting the entire package — development of faculty, clinical programs, cooperation of the hospitals, space, and equipment — together."[27]

INTO THE FUTURE

AT PRESENT NEARLY 25 percent of practicing optometrists are nearing or at retirement age. Over 130 million Americans are already wearing corrective eyewear, plus the U.S. has a growing and aging population which includes an estimated 61 million people in need of vision care. Asked about this probable increase in the demand for optometrists in the near future, Banwell replied: "Whether there are a lot of patients and a few doctors, or just the opposite, isn't really an issue here. No matter what, there will always be a demand for the best trained, most highly-skilled professionals. Those will be the success stories of tomorrow."

Maintaining the leadership position in optometric education, and incorporating computerization into educational programs along with other technological advances which improve primary eye care services have become imperative goals for ICO's administration. In an assessment of ICO's current and future academic and clinical needs a second 10-year plan has been designed.

The range of the IEI's health care services are being expanded to provide interdisciplinary experiences for the student body, and enhanced primary medical care services for the community. Soon to be added is a program based within Illinois Masonic Medical Center that will include 10 full-time ICO examination rooms, providing the school with a greater north-side community presence. (Presently, ICO has student training programs at Illinois Masonic's main hospital facility and in one of its primary care satellite facilities.)

The success of IEI's binocular vision/pediatric care service has warranted plans for additional examination and consultation rooms. Special testing areas have been allocated for oculomotor and electrophysiology; photorefraction; preferential visual acuity; preferential stereopsis and contrast sensitivity; and visual fields instrumentation geared for testing infants and toddlers.

The Easter Seal Society program's growth has also made it necessary to increase the number of designated examination rooms; adding another consultation room; and constructing a self-contained waiting area for these special patients. It is hoped this particular effort will establish a national model for multi-handicapped patient eye care service.

Providing better patient care and higher quality education, improved patient facilities in these areas will enhance both primary and pediatric care clinical research. Laboratory facilities designed to incorporate new computer-oriented learning techniques such as a self-paced learning systems through the use of computer-generated anatomical sections (and similarly enhanced techniques applied to other teaching areas) are also in the planning stages.

The recently renovated IEI clinic amphitheater (The Adams Center for Clinical Learning) improves the ratio of student-observations to live patient care activities occurring in the advanced ophthalmic care service areas without intruding on patient privacy by the application of improved audio-visual technologies. This configuration enhances the effectiveness and efficiency of continuing education programs and "grand rounds" presentations.

In order to handle existing and future space requirements — and to house a up to 640 students on campus — ICO, in collaboration with Knight Architects Engineers Planners Inc., has developed a comprehensive plan for renovating some of the existing facilities and building essential new components. The construction of the new 200-student, 70,000 square-foot on-campus residential complex with student lounges, storage, and laundry facilities is replacing Brady Hall. On the site of Brady Hall, a new 50,000-square-foot clinic building addition will be dedicated to pediatric care, clinic administration, and teaching laboratories. In the existing IEI building, approximately 25,000-square-feet will be renovated to accommodate additional clinic and research facilities, further increasing IEI's efficiency in patient care.

ICO continues its commitment to helping graduates establish themselves as practitioners, and helping practitioners update and improve their existing skills. Since its inception in 1991, ICO's Professional Placement Program has not only matched graduates with goal-oriented positions, they have also served as liaison between private practitioners and future associates or potential buyers.

OVER THE PAST 125 years, the optometric profession and ICO have grown side by side, offering unique opportunities to practitioners, students, and educators for personal and professional fulfillment. Optometry has truly emerged as an essential and cost-effective part of the nation's health care system. Optometric practitioners will never have to struggle for recognition as a profession or for the right to provide patients with care again. Their predecessors have championed those battles. The challenges facing future optometrists are directly related to improving eye care through the discovery of new cures and preventive measures; and making sure optometric services are available to everyone who needs them in the new millennia.

The history of the schools who have been chronicled in this book has also been an integral part of so many professionals' lives. ICO is very proud of the roles its graduates have played in the profession's growth, and looks forward to many years of continued participation — contributing to optometry's future. And as inconceivable as it may be, the next century will undoubtedly be even more eventful.

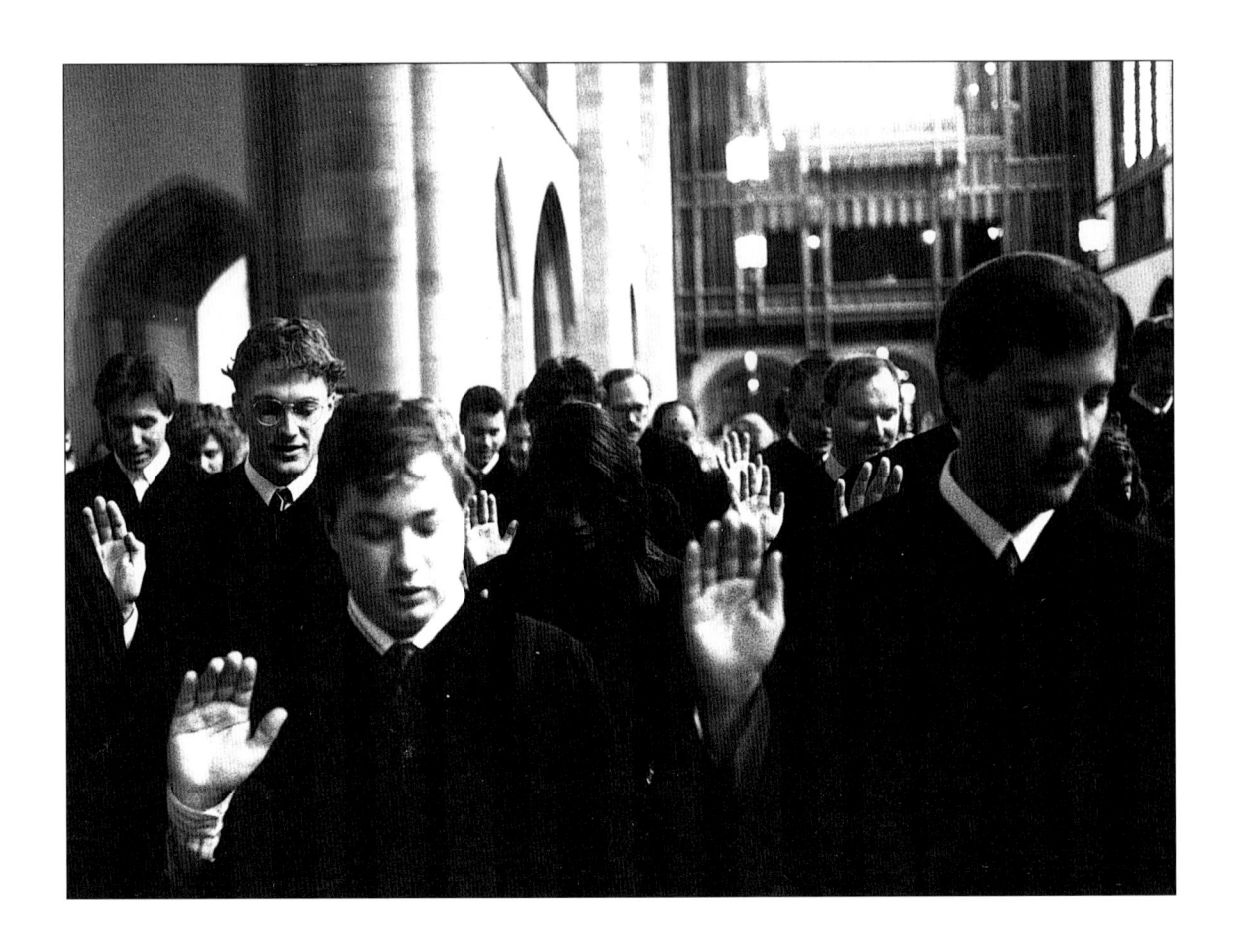

1783 – James McAllister reputedly opens the first optical shop in Philadelphia, PA.

1784 – Benjamin Franklin designs a bicentric lens system for his own use.

1803 – Karl Himley begins teaching ophthalmology as a special discipline in Göttingen, Germany.

1847 – British astronomer and lensmaker Charles Babbage invents the Babbage ophthalmoscope.

1848 – The American Medical Association (AMA) is founded.

1850 – Ophthalmology becomes a full-blown specialty when a number of hospitals dedicated to the treatment of eye diseases emerge in Great Britain and America.

1851 – Hermann Ludwig Ferdinand von Helmholz, a Prussian physicist and physiologist, invents an ophthalmoscope and publishes his results.

1862 – James Burton McFatrich is born in Lena, Illinois.

1864 – The American Ophthalmological Society is founded in New York.

1866 – von Helmholz develops an ophthalmometer and publishes *Physiological Optics*.

1872 – Dr. Henry Olin founds the Chicago College of Ophthalmology and Otology.

1878 – Charles A. Spencer, a New York microscope maker, wins the Paris Exposition's Gold Medal.
– Dr. Olin incorporates the Chicago College of Ophthalmology and Otology.

1879 – James Burton McFatrich enrolls in both Hahnemann Medical College and Bennett College of Medicine and Surgery.
– William Bray Needles is born in Sedalia, Missouri.

1887 – Dr. James McFatrich joins Dr. Olin as a full partner in a practice specializing ophthalmology, after a 2-year Cook County Hospital internship. He joins Olin's faculty.

1888 – The first contact lenses are simultaneously developed by Dr. A. Eugen Fick in Switzerland and by Edouard Kalt, a Parisian spectaclemaker.

1889 – Dr. Olin retires for health reasons, and Dr. McFatrich takes over both the practice and the school's management.

1891 – Dr. Olin dies. Dr. McFatrich assumes complete control of the school, changes the institution's name to Northern Illinois College of Ophthalmology and Otology (NICOO).

1892 – Charles F. Prentice of New York replies to Dr. Henry D. Noyes who has reprimanded him for charging a professional fee for advising an optical patient.
– Dr. McFatrich's brother George Wilbur McFatrich completes his training at Bennett College and becomes a Cook County Hospital house physician.

1893 – Dr. Charles McCormick establishes the McCormick Optical College in Chicago.
– Dr. George W. McFatrich is appointed attending surgeon and oculist. He is also elected as Professor of Ophthalmology and Otology at Bennett College. He then joins the NICOO staff.

1896 – Drs. Charles F. Prentice and Andrew J. Cross along with other New York practitioners organize The Optical Society of the State of New York.
– The McFatriches incorporate NICOO.

1897 – The McFatriches establish the Murine Eye Remedy Company along with Otis F. Hall.

1898 – Reuben Seid is born.
– Dr. Andrew Jay Cross is elected president of the New York State Society of Optometrists.
– Dr. George McFatrich takes over most of NICOO's management and amends the school's charter to include the admission of non-medical candidates.
– Great Britain's Worshipful Company of Spectaclemakers institutes periodic re-certification examinations for practicing refractionists.
– The first gathering of charter members in the American Association of Opticians meets in New York City.

1899 – William Bray Needles attends classes at Chicago's McCormick Optical College.

1900 – Dr. Andrew Jay Cross becomes the first optometrist elected as

CHRONOLOGY

129

president of the American Optical Association.

1901 – The state of Minnesota passes the first laws regulating optometric practice, licensing and education.

1903 – Dr. Needles conducts a series of successful evening optometric lectures and workshops, and teaches refracting courses sponsored by the F.C. Merry Company while teaching at the Kansas City School of Optometry.

1904 – The American Association of Opticians votes a woman into the post of second vice-president.
– The AMA's Council on Education standardizes both the entry requirements and the curriculum taught in U.S. medical schools.

1906 – The American Association of Opticians adds nearly 800 new members to its original roster of 183.

1907 – Dr. Needles founds the Needles Institute of Optometry.
– The American Association of Optician's Physiological Section appoint a female vice president.

1908 – The American Association of Opticians adopts a Code of Ethics.
– The Illinois state legislature passes an optometric bill.

1910 – Dr. Needles incorporates his school.
– Columbia University becomes the first American university to offer optometry courses.

1912 – Dr. William Bates is dropped from AMA membership because of his vision training theories.
– The American Association of Opticians Education Committee's requisite cirriculum is adopted.

1914 – Dr. James B. McFatrich dies.
– State optometric laws added further educational requirements.

1915 – Ohio State University adds a 4-year undergraduate optometric course.
– The National Organization of State Boards of Examiners in Optometry adopt the American Association of Optician's curriculum.
– Dr. Needles gives a week-long seminar at the University of California at Berkeley, part of a natonwide lecture tour.

1917 – Dr. Charles Sheard publishes his 18-point testing technique entitled *Dynamic Ocular Tests*.

– Dr. George McFatrich resigns as the NICOO's president and secretary, but still maintains controlling interest in the school's stock.
– The United States enters the First World War.

1918 – The International Association of Boards of Examiners in Optometry standardizes schools' admissions policies and curriculum.

1919 – The American Association of Opticians changes its name to the American Optometric Association (AOA).

1920 – Researchers discover that human vision is not only optically-based, but is also a physiological function.
– Dr. William Bates publishes his Bates Method theories fostering further interest in vision training (orthoptics) by optometrists.

1921 – During a Chicago speaking engagement Dr. William Needles meets with Dr. George McFatrich, who offers him ownership of NICOO.

1922 – Needles purchases NICOO's outstanding stock. He leaves Dr. Ernest Occhiena in charge of the Needles Institute of Optometry.
– Thirty out of 60 independent U.S. optometry schools remain in operation.

1923 – Dr. Carl F. Shepard heads NICOO's research department.
– The University of California at Berkeley starts its own 4-year program.

1924 – The District of Columbia becomes the last continental territory to pass an optometric bill.

1926 – Dr. Reuben Seid graduates in 1926 from the University of Illinois.
– NICOO moves from the Masonic Temple Building to Drexel Blvd.

1926 – Dr. A.M. Skeffington establishes NICOO summer courses.
– Dr. Needles merges his schools, moves operations to Chicago, and changes the school's name to Northern Illinois College of Optometry (NICO).

1928 – The Alpha Chapter of Phi Kappa Rho, an optometric sorority, is founded at NICO.

1929 – The Great Depression begins a general economic downturn that lasts for nearly a decade.

1930 – Polaroid markets sun glasses.
– The AMA Council on Education warns medical schools against admitting too many students. They also encourage state licensing boards to adopt tougher regulations on immigrating physicians.
– Dr. A.M. Skeffington establishes the Optometric Extension Program in Oklahoma.
– Dr. Carl F. Shepard develops the Keystone stereoscope.
– NICO adds a 2000-hour/2-year Doctor of Optometry degree to the curriculum.

1931 – NICO's Dr. W. D. Zoethout publishes his book, *Physiology*.

1932 – Northern Illinois Eye Clinic begins treating patients from the surrounding schools and welfare agencies.

1933 – Needles changes his admission policies and curriculum.

1934 – Needles announces an expansion of both NICO's faculty, curriculum, and physical plant.

1936 – Dr. Seid establishes the Midwestern College of Optometry.
– NICO opens its first dormitory.
– The AMA institutes a gag rule that prohibits ophthalmologists from lecturing at optometric institutions.
– The first plastic contact lenses are developed by Dr. William Feinbloom, a Manhattan optometrist.

1937 – Dr. Seid hires Dr. Carl Shepard from NICO to serve as dean and renames his school the Monroe College of Optometry (MCO).
– Morton Abram graduates from De Paul University Law School.

1938 – John Mullen and Theodore Obrig discover that hard contact lenses can be made from polymethyl methacrylate (PMMA).
– NICO adds a fourth year to its curriculum.

1940 – Dr. Eugene Strawn graduates from MCO as class valedictorian.
– The AOA authorizes the American Women's Optometric Association.

1941 – MCO moves to a building near the Chicago River.
– MCO offers a 4-year optometric course.
– The International Board of Boards (IBB) gives MCO's curriculum a Class A rating.

– The AOA adopts the *Manual of Accrediting Schools and Colleges of Optometry* written by NICO's Drs. Irvin Borish and Eugene Freeman.

1944 – The AOA enhances their Code of Ethics.
– The U.S. Congress passes the G.I. Bill of Rights.

1945 – MCO moves to the Owen Building on Larrabee Street.
– Morton Abram becomes MCO's Assistant Director.
– The U.S. federal government creates an Optometry Section in the Army-Navy Medical Corps.

1946 – A supplement to the AOA Code of Ethics is added.

1947 – Dr. Eugene Freeman becomes dean of MCO.
– Dr. James Grout becomes NICO's Clinic Director.
– Kevin Tuohy develops the corneal contact lens.
– Morton Abram changes MCO's name to Chicago College of Optometry (CCO) and files a Council on Education accreditation application.

1947 – The number of practicing optometrists in the U.S. falls to its lowest point in modern history.

1948 – CCO moves to a new campus near Clark and Belden Streets.
– CCO students take part in the Chicago Strabismus Project.
– Dr. Carl Shepard heads the revival of NICO's research department.
– Dr. William B. Needles dies.
– NICO hires Dr. Howard Egan as dean.
– The Northern Illinois Eye Clinic expands its facilities.

1949 – CCO establishes itself with a full 5-year course.
– CCO appoints its first Clinic Administrator, Dr. Ernest S. Takahashi.
– The first African-American optometrist to become a faculty member at an accredited U.S. college, Dr. Junius Brodnax, joins the CCO staff.
– Dr. Walter Yasko becomes Northern Illinois Eye Clinic's assistant chief of staff.

1950 – CCO receives its full accreditation.
– Dr. Eugene Tennant becomes CCO's Clinic Administrator.

– Dr. Frederick Kushner is appointed NICO's dean.
– Dr. Thaddeus Murroughs becomes CCO's research director.
– The AMA lifts their gag rule that prohibits ophthalmologists from lecturing at optometric institutions.
– William Needles' son, Dr. Richard Needles is appointed NICO president.

1951 – Dr. Reuben Seid dies from a heart attack.
– Dr. Richard Feinberg becomes NICO's president.
– Morton Abram becomes CCO's president.

1952 – Dr. Eugene Strawn becomes president of CCO's Alumni Association. He soon becomes a board member and its executive vice-president.

1953 – NICO starts offering student loans.

1954 – The groundbreaking ceremony for CCO's new building takes place; and the fall session opens at the new school.

1955 – Dr. Eugene Strawn becomes CCO's president.
– Dr. Eugene Strawn becomes ICO's president.
– Dr. Yasko replaces Dr. Eugene Tennant as NICO's clinic director.
– NICO and CCO merge to become Illinois College of Optometry (ICO).
– Dr. Alfred A. Rosenbloom, Jr., becomes ICO's dean.
– Dr. Frederick Kushner becomes ICO's Alumni Association president.

1956 – The ICO Eye Clinic is dedicated.

1958 – ICO starts student externship program.

1959 – Dr. Leo Manas invents the ICO Maze.

1961 – Dr. C.K. Hill joins Dr. Kushner in Alumi Association fund raising drive.

1963 – Optometry is included in the federal Health Professions Educational Assistance Act of 1963.

1964 – Ground is broken for Brady Hall.

1965 – Brady Hall is dedicated and ground is broken for a clinic wing.
– Optometry is included in the government's 1965 list of Medicaid services.

1967 – The OEO and HEW launch 150 neighborhood health centers as part of a federal program.
– ICO changes its curriculum from a 3-year to a 4-year professional program.

1968 – The AOA's Department of National Affairs reports that numerous federal agencies are employing full-time and consulting optometrists.

1969 – Dr. Strawn appoints ICO registrar Dr. Jess E. Goroshow to the new post of assistant to the president.

1971 – Dr. Strawn dies in Toronto.
– Board chairman Dr. O.W. Weinstein becomes ICO interim president.
– The state of Rhode Island enacts legislation permitting optometrists to use DPAs.

1972 – Dr. Alfred A. Rosenbloom, Jr. becomes ICO president.
– Dr. Earl P. Fisher is elected board chairman, and board member Dr. Boyd Banwell becomes vice-chair.
– Dr. Peter Nelson and some of his ICO students independently launch the Vision Project.
– ICO celebrates its centennial
– ICO establishes a "Promise to Go Back" scholarship to fund students who pledge to work in minority neighborhoods after graduation.

1973 – National Optometric Association honors ICO as College of the Year.

1974 – Dr. Boyd Banwell is elected board chairman.

1975 – ICO acquires a VER computer through a National Eye Institute grant.

1977 – ICO's infant care clinic opens.
– Four ICO students participate in the Volunteer Optometric Services to Humanity (VOSH) program.

1978 – Dr. Anthony Nizza becomes ICO Eye Clinic's first Residency Program director.
– Federal Health Services and Centers Amendments of 1978 describes optometrists as "best suited by training and practice to deliver primary care vision services."

1981 – Dr. Rosenbloom resigns his position as ICO's president and becomes the school's first Distinguished Professor of Optometry.
– Dr. Fredrick R. Kushner becomes board chairman, and Dr. Joseph L. Henry becomes chairman-elect.

- Dr. Boyd B. Banwell becomes interim ICO president.
1982 – ICO adopts a renewable contract tenure system.
- Banwell becomes ICO president.
1983 – Sports Vision service established.
- Dr. Joseph L. Henry becomes board chairman, and Dr. Joseph Ebbeson becomes chairman-elect.
1984 – Dr. David A. Greenberg appointed Vice President for Academic Affairs and Dean.
- ICO Eye Clinic is renamed Illinois Eye Institute (IEI).
1985 – 50,000 sq. ft. building addition completed.
1987 – Dr. W. Judd Chapman becomes board chairman.
1988 – COE awards ICO maximum professional accreditation.
- Strawn Wing ground floor completed.
1989 – North Central Association of Schools and Colleges awards ICO maximum accreditation.
1991 – IEI-Easter Seals Eye Care Program established.
- IEI established 24-hour walk-in emergency vision care service.
- Ebbeson becomes board chairman; and Dr. A. Rodriguez becomes chairman-elect.
1994 – ICO offers nation's first combined O.D./Ph.D. degree program.
1995 – Illinois Senate Bill 185 allows certified Illinois optometrists to use TPAs.
- Illinois Optometric Practice Act amendment allows "as taught" legislation.

THE BOARD OF TRUSTEES

Dr. John E. Brandt
Dr. James R. Butler
Dr. W. Judd Chapman
Dr. Joseph B. Ebbeson
Dr. Joseph L. Henry
Dr. C.K. Hill
Dr. Frederick R. Kushner
Mrs. Nancy Philip
Dr. Ward R. Ransdell
Dr. Albert H. Rodriguez, Jr.
Mr. Benjamin S. Wolfe
Dr. Howard I. Woolf

ALUMNI COUNCIL MEMBERS

Dr. John E. Brandt
Dr. James R. Butler *
Dr. Brian W. Caden
Dr. Tony Q. Chan *
Dr. Thaddeus S. Depukat
Dr. Albert H. Eschen
Dr. Earl P. Fisher
Dr. Seymour Galina
Dr. James Gardner
Dr. James B. Hasler *
Dr. Richard F. Hickman
Dr. C.K. Hill
Dr. Richard G. Jarvis
Dr. Louis J. Katz
Dr. Phillip L. Kaufman
Dr. Michael Kotlicky
Dr. Frederick R. Kushner
Dr. Gary W. Lasken *
Dr. Lori Latowski Grover *
Dr. Frank Lazovick
Dr. Kenneth P. Martin

Dr. Donald Mazzula
Dr. Norman G. Michaud
Dr. Paul D. Randolph
Dr. Ward R. Ransdell
Dr. Janice Scharre
Dr. Martin J. Sikorski *
Dr. James A. Stewart
Dr. Lawrence R. Vogel
Dr. Wendell D. Waldie
Dr. Howard I. Woolf

*   *Present Council members*

NOTE:
   This information was derived from Alumni Council Members and Graduation Years list.

AOA PRESIDENTS

The following AOA presidents graduated or took post-graduate courses at either Illinois College of Optometry (ICO) or its predecessor schools: Northern Illinois College of Ophthalmology and Otology (NICOO), Northern Illinois College of Optometry (NICO), Needles Institute of Optometry, .

John C. Eberhardt (1903)
   NICOO, 1898 and 1899

Briggs S. Palmer (1906 – 1907)
   Needles Institute of Optometry

Chester N. McDonnell (1910)
   Needles Institute of Optometry

George L. Schneider (1911)
   Chicago College of Ophthalmology and Otology, 1897

William S. Todd (1922)
   NICO, 1901, and Needles Institute of Optometry, 1919

Thomas H. Martin (1923 – 1924)
   Needles Institute of Optometry

Walter F. Kimball (1925 – 1926)
   Needles Institute of Optometry

Harry E. Pine (1936 – 1937)
   NICO, 1920, 1923, and 1932

Ewing Adams (1942 – 1943)
   Needles Institute of Optometry, 1914

William Carey Ezell (1944 – 1945)
   NICO, 1917

James Fredreick Wahl (1952 – 1953)
   Needles Institute of Optometry, 1923, and NICO

Leslie Holman Sugarman (1957)
   NICO, 1933

Phinehas.N. DeVere (1959)
   NICO, 1932 and 1934

Richard C. Schiller (1960)
   NICO, 1939

Don Abell Frantz (1961)
   NICO, 1937

W. Judd Chapman (1963)
   NICO, 1949

Vernon Eugene McCrary (1965)
   NICO, 1949

John G. Sugg (1967)
   NICO, 1949

James C. Tumblin (1972)
   NICO, 1948

Bernard J. Shannon (1974)
   ICO, 1952 and 1956

Howard P. Winton (1975)
   NICO, 1949

Jack W. Von Bokern (1980)
   NICO, 1951

Wendell D. Waldie (1982)
   NICO, 1949

Albert A. Bucar (1984)
   ICO, 1954 and 1955

James C. Leadingham (1992)
   ICO, 1965

NOTE: Information derived from Presidents of American Optometric Association Graduated from Illinois College of Optometry, compiled by ILAMO, 1987 (updated, Mar 1996); and AOA Presidents — Education, 1992.

HONORARY DEGREES

(Doctor of Ocular Science (DOS), Doctor of Human Letters in Optometry (LHD))

1954 Joseph Tiffin, Ph.D. (DOS)

1955 Marguerite T. Eberl, O.D. (DOS)
Malcolm E. Edwards, O.D. (DOS)
Felix Koetting, O.D. (DOS)

1956 John R. Kennedy, O.D. (DOS)

1959 William Scott Gray, Ph.D. (DOS)

1961 Kenneth P. Martin, O.D. (DOS)
Henry E. Quick, O.D. (DOS)
John G. Sugg, O.D. (DOS)

1963 Dr. H. Ewalt, Jr. (DOS)
Leonard Shanfield, B.S.L., L.L.B. (LHD)

1964 M.E. Broom, Ph.D. (DOS)
W. Clement Stone (LHD)
Roy Paul Stealey (LHD)

1966 Dr. W. Judd Chapman (DOS)
Dr. Princhas Neilds DeVere (DOS)
Dr. Walter S. Yasko (DOS)
J. Harold Bailey (LHD)
Dr. Ellen Louise Colley (LHD)

1968 Dr. Ernest B. Alexander (DOS)
Dr. Lawrence Fitch (DOS)
Dr. Meredith Walter Morgan (DOS)

1969 Brigadier General William A. Hamrick, U.S.A., M.S.C., Chief Service Corps, U.S. Army (DOS)
Capt. Robert S. Hermann, U.S.N. (DOS)
Col. Alvin F. Meyer, Jr., U.S.A.F. (DOS)
The Honorable Paul Powell (LHD)

1972 Dr. V. Eugene McCrary (DOS)
Dr. Robert F. Jamieson (DOS)
Dr. Jess T. Goroshow (DOS)

1973 Dr. Seymour Galina (DOS)
Albert E. Schoenbeck (LHD)
Dr. Joseph Louis Henry (LHD)

1974 Dr. Earl P. Fisher (DOS)
Dr. Edward Scanlan (DOS)
Dr. J.C. Tumblin (DOS)

1975 Dr. Bernard Grolman (DOS)
Dr. Charles E. Seger (DOS)

1976 Charles Eric Bateman, F.B.O.A., H.D., D.Orth. (DOS)
Ruth Penrod Morris, O.D. (DOS)
Albert N. Lemoine, Jr., A.B., M.D., F.A.C.S. (LHD)

1977 John Logan Howlette, O.D. (DOS)

1978 Dr. Boyd B. Banwell (DOS)
Dr. Joseph B. Ebbesen (DOS)

1979 Dr. Monroe J. Hirsch (DOS)
Samuel M. Genensky, Ph.D. (LHD)

1980 The Honorable James R. Thompson, Governor of the State of Illinois (DOS)

1981 The Honorable Robert Whittaker, O.D., F.A.A.O. (DOS)

1982 Eleanor E. Faye, A.B., M.D. (LHD)

1984 Wendell Waldie, O.D. (DOS)

1985 Albert A. Bucar, O.D. (DOS)
Wilhelm Joachim Pohl, O.D., M.D. (DOS)

1986 C. Clayton Powell, O.D., M.P.H. (DOS)

1988 Earle L. Hunter, O.D., C.A.E. (DOS)
Virgil W. Deering (LHD)

1989 David Greenberg, O.D., M.P.H. (DOS)
Shane J. Conway (LHD)

1990 Benjamin S. Wolfe, (LHD)
Melvin D. Wolfberg, O.D. (DOS)

1992 Louis J. Katz, O.D. (DOS)
Hyman S. Wodis, O.D. (posthumous) (DOS)
Awarded for more than 50 years of service to the profession and ICO.

1993 Thaddeus S. Depukat, O.D., F.A.A.O., F.C.O.V.D. (DOS)
James C. Leadingham, O.D., F.A.A.O. (DOS)

1994 John E. Brandt, O.D. (DOS)

1995 Howard I. Woolf, O.D. F.A.A.O. (DOS)

ALUMNI ASSOCIATION AWARD RECIPIENTS

Lifetime Service Award

1992 Fred Kushner, O.D., D.O.S.
1993 C.K. Hill, O.D., D.O.S.
1994 Joseph Ebbesen, O.D.

DISTINGUISHED ALUMNUS

1993 Albert Eschen, O.D.
     Yale Knight, O.D.
1994 Wilhelm Pohl, O.D.
1995 James B. Hasler, O.D.

ALUMNUS/ALUMNA OF THE YEAR

1972 Alfred Rosenbloom, Jr., O.D.
1973 C.K. Hill, O.D.
1974 Kenneth Martin, O.D.
1975 W. Judd Chapman, O.D.
1976 Sylvio Dupuis, O.D.
1977 Franklin Harms, O.D.
1978 Robert Jamieson, O.D.
1979 John Janney, O.D.
1980 Donald Heyden, O.D.
1981 Jess E. Goroshow, O.D.
1982 Floyd D. Mizener, O.D.
1983 Norman G. Michaud, O.D.
1984 Burton Skuza, O.D.
1985 James C. Leadingham, O.D.
1986 Wendell D. Waldie, O.D.
1987 Robert R. Whittaker, O.D.
1988 Boyd B. Banwell, O.D.
1989 James R. Butler, O.D.
1990 Brian Klinger, O.D.
1991 Robert Johnson, O.D.
1992 Louis Katz, O.D.
1993 Janice Scharre, O.D.
1994 Janice M. Jurkus, O.D.

NOTE: Information derived from Office of the Registrar Honorary Degrees list; and Alumni Association Award Recipients list.

In citing works in these notes, the following abbreviations have been used for frequently cited journals, books and authors:

AJO	*The American Journal of Optics*
AOA	American Optometric Association
cat.	school catalog
CCO	Chicago College of Optometry
CHGO	Chicago, IL
Focus	Reprint of "Focus on the Future: Illinois College of Optometry," JAOA 43:5 (May 1972)
Glasses	Drs. Alvin and Virginia B. Silverstein, *Glasses and Contact Lenses: Your Guide to Eyes, Eyewear, and Eye Care* (NYC: J.B. Lippincott, 19??)
ICO	Illinois College of Optometry
IL OP	The Illinois Optometrist
JAOA	*The Journal of the American Optometric Association*
NICO	Northern Illinois College of Optometry
NICOO	Northern Illinois College of Ophthalmology and Otology
NYC	New York City, New York
OJ	*The Optical Journal*
OJ&RO	*The Optical Journal and Review of Optometry*
Optometry	Maurice A. Cox, *Optometry: The Profession, Its Antecedents, Birth and Development* (PHIL: Chilton Book Co., 1947)
Opt. Prof.	Drs. Monroe J. Hirsch, O.D. and Ralph E. Wick, O.D., D.O.S., *The Optometric Profession* (Philadelphia, PA: Chilton Book Co., 1968)
OR	*The Optical Review*
OW	*The Optometric Weekly*
St.L	St. Louis, MO

CHAPTER ONE

1. Dr. James R. Gregg, O.D., *The Story of Optometry* (NYC: Ronald Press, 1965) 41-43; *Optometry* 5.
2. *Opt. Prof.* 46 and 56-57.
3. Ibid. 67-68 and 71; Dr. James R. Gregg, O.D., *The Story of Optometry* (NYC: Ronald Press, 1965) 10 and 31-32.
4. In historical accounts of Chinese emperor Pu Yi's life during the 1900s, there is a story that when it was discovered that Pu Yi was myopic, the court objected to the suggestion that he had to wear spectacles based on the fact it was a sign of weakness. See also *Opt. Prof.* 68; *Glasses* 6; Dr. L.D. Bronson, *Early American Specs: An Exciting Collectible* (Glendale, CA: The Occidental Publishing Co., 1974) 20; Dr. James R. Gregg, O.D., *The Story of Optometry* (NYC: Ronald Press, 1965) 50-51 and 52; *Optometry* 3; "Ancient Chinese Eye-Care," IL OP (Jul-Aug 1954) 16.
5. Dr. James R. Gregg, O.D., *The Story of Optometry* (NYC: Ronald Press, 1965) 47 and 49; *Opt. Prof.* 70, 73-75; Dr. L.D. Bronson, *Early American Specs: An Exciting Collectible*. (Glendale, CA: The Occidental Publishing Co., 1974) 22; *Optometry* 4.
6. *Opt. Prof.* 79; *Glasses* 9; Dr. James R. Gregg, O.D., *The Story of Optometry* (NYC: Ronald Press, 1965) 53.
7. *Opt. Prof.* 79; *Glasses* 9; Dr. James R. Gregg, O.D., *The Story of Optometry* (NYC: Ronald Press, 1965) 53.
8. *Optometry* 3.
9. Fred L. Pick and G. Norman Knight, rev. by Frederick Smith, *The Pocket History of Freemasonry* (London (UK): Hutchinson, 1953, rev. 1992) 19-23.
10. Ibid.
11. *Opt. Prof.* 81; Dr. James R. Gregg, O.D., *The Story of Optometry* (NYC: Ronald Press, 1965) 58.
12. *Opt. Prof.* 82 and 85.
13. Paul Starr, *The Social Transformation of American Medicine*. (NYC: Basic Books, 1982) 37-38 and 43.
14. According to H.W. Hofstetter, *Optometry: Professional, Economic, and Legal Aspects* (St.L: The C.V. Mosby Co., 1948) 279, The Master and Court of the Worshipful Co. of Spectaclemakers was chartered by King Charles I of England in 1629 and ratified by an Act of Parliament in 1690.
See also *Opt. Prof.* 84; Dr. James R. Gregg, O.D., *The Story of Optometry* (NYC: Ronald Press, 1965) 58.
15. According to Dr. James R. Gregg, O.D., *The Story of Optometry* (NYC: Ronald Press, 1965) 60 the government at Nuremberg was forced by the pressures of the Regensberg free guild of spectaclemakers to regulated the sale of Venetian spectacles. Only lens peddlers could sell the imported lenses while shopkeepers were limited to selling locally-produced products.
See also *Opt. Prof.* 82-83 and 86.
16. *Opt. Prof.* 82.
17. Ibid. 87.
18. Bartisch, a member of the barber-surgeon guild in Saxony, Germany had become an oculist later in his career.
See also *Opt. Prof.* 77-78; Dr. L.D. Bronson, *Early American Specs: An Exciting Collectible* (Glendale, CA: The Occidental Publishing Co., 1974) 28; Dr. Sidney Groffman, O.D., D.O.S. "The Eyes of Liberty," JAOA 47:8 (Aug 1976)1034.
19. Dr. James R. Gregg, O.D., *The Story of Optometry* (NYC: Ronald Press, 1965) 61-63; *Optometry* 8.
20. Dr. Sidney Groffman, O.D., D.O.S. "The Eyes of Liberty," JAOA 47:8 (Aug 1976) 1034.
21. Ibid.
22. See also Dr. Sidney Groffman, O.D., D.O.S. "The Eyes of Liberty," JAOA 47:8 (Aug 1976) 1034 and 1021; *Opt. Prof.* 126; Dr. James R. Gregg, O.D., *The Story of Optometry* (NYC: Ronald Press, 1965) 136 and 161.
23. Dr. Sidney Groffman, O.D., D.O.S. "The Eyes of Liberty," JAOA 47:8 (Aug 1976) 1038-1039.
24. Ibid.; Dr. James R. Gregg, O.D., *The Story of Optometry* (NYC: Ronald Press, 1965) 147 and 161.
25. H.W. Hofstetter, *Optometry: Professional, Economic, and Legal Aspects* (St.L: The C.V. Mosby Co., 1948) 354; Paul Starr, *The Social Transformation of American Medicine*. (NYC: Basic Books, 1982) 6-7 and 30-31.
26. Oculist is an archane term used to define an optometrist during the late nineteenth-century.
27. *Opt. Prof.* 127.
28. Ibid.;E.E. Arrington *History of Optometry* (CHGO: White Printing House, 1929) 16.
29. Dr. James R. Gregg, O.D., *The Story of Optometry* (NYC: Ronald Press, 1965) 165.
30. *Opt. Prof.* 126-127; *Optometry* 19-20.
31. *Optometry* 6; Dr. James R. Gregg, O.D., *The Story of Optometry* (NYC: Ronald Press, 1965) 100-101.
32. Dr. James R. Gregg, O.D., *The Story of Optometry* (NYC: Ronald Press, 1965) 102-104

NOTES

and 293; *Optometry* 6; E.E. Arrington *History of Optometry* (CHGO: White Printing House, 1929) 15.
33. Dr. James R. Gregg, O.D., *The Story of Optometry* (NYC: Ronald Press, 1965) 174.
34. Ibid. 162-163; *Optometry* 11.
35. Dr. James R. Gregg, O.D., *The Story of Optometry* (NYC: Ronald Press, 1965) 166-168; *Optometry* 15; E.E. Arrington *History of Optometry* (CHGO: White Printing House, 1929) 119-120.

CHAPTER TWO

1. Lewis Osborne, *The Great Chicago Fire of 1871: Three Illustrated Accounts from Harper's Weekly.* (Ashland, IL: Lewis Osborne, 1969) 7 and 54.
2. Dr. James R. Gregg, O.D. *The Story of Optometry* (NYC: The Ronald Press, 1965) 275.
3. *Biographical Dictionary and Portrait Gallery of Chicago* 390-395.
4. Chartered in 1895 Hahnemann Medical College and Bennett Medical College (chartered in 1868) had hospital facilities for the clinical training of students. Eventually Hahnemann merged with Chicago Homeopathic College to teach homeopathy which relied Nicholas Culpepper's theories and other early herbal healers. Bennett College taught Eclectic medicine which taught that it is the patient, not the disease that should be treated.
See also *The United States Biographical Dictionary, 1890* 223-224; *History of Chicago and Cook County,* 1912 315-316.
5. *Polk's Medical and Surgical Register of the United States* (Detroit, MI: R.L. Polk & Co., Publishers, 1893) 284; *Focus* 4.
6. According to *Polk's Medical and Surgical Register of the United States* (Detroit, MI: R.L. Polk & Co., Publishers, 1893) 1369, the Chicago Ophthalmic College was incorporated in 1886 by Dr. H.M. Martin, P.C., M.D. A short account this school can be found in "Your Classmates," Optometry (Jun 1915). See also *Optometry* 31; Dr. James R. Gregg, O.D. *The Story of Optometry* (NYC: The Ronald Press, 1965) 219; and H.W. Hofstetter, *Optometry: Professional, Economic, and Legal Aspects* (St.L: The C.V. Mosby Co., 1948) 297.
7. *Biographical Dictionary and Portrait Gallery of Chicago* 390-395; *Focus* 4.
For an account of the Masonic Temple Building see John J. Flinn, *Chicago: The Marvelous City of the West—A History, An Encyclopedia, and Guide (2nd ed.)* (CHGO: The Standard Guide Co., 1892) 583-585.
8. *Focus* 4; "Northern Illinois College of Ophthalmology and Otology," OJ 15:9 (Feb 23 1905) 428.
9. Letter to Wm. Greenberg from Dr. G.W. McFatrich (Sep 28 1917).
10. "The Northern Illinois College of Ophthalmology and Otology," OJ 15:9 (Feb 23 1905) 425; State of Illinois Certificate of Incorporation issued to the Northern Illinois College of Ophthalmology (Feb 26 1896).
11. For a short history of the invention of Murine and the the relationship between the McFatrich brothers and Otis Hall see Sir Knight Thomas Regis, M.P.S., "The Doctors McFatrich," *Knight Templar* 29:8 (Aug 1983) 23-26.
12. Dr. James B. McFatrich, "Deplorable Conditions," OJ 10:1 (Jul 1902) 82-83.
13. Ibid.; .Dr. James R. Gregg, O.D. *The Story of Optometry* (NYC: The Ronald Press, 1965) 191 and 220.
One of NICOO's faculty, Professor E.G. Trowbridge also contributed an article "License for Opticians," OJ 10:1 (Jul 1902) 75, which called for opticians to be educated and licensed in the same manner as physicians and dentists.
14. *Focus* 4; "Announcement," *Northern Illinois College of Ophthalmology and Otology* (cat., CHGO: NICOO, 1909).
The school justified education in refraction to both medical and non-medical applicants in "For Jewelers, Druggists, Physicians," *Northern Illinois College of Ophthalmology and Otology* (cat., CHGO: NICOO, 1909). An account of a simple practice room can be found in Dr. H.A. Thomson, "Dr. Thomson's Correspondence Course in Optics: Lesson #15," (H.A. Thomson, 1895) 1-3.
15. According to Dr. James R. Gregg, O.D. *The Story of Optometry* (NYC: The Ronald Press, 1965) 170-171, The Spencer Optical Manufacturing Co. was renamed in 1895 to the Spencer Lens Co. In 1935, the American Optical Co. acquired the company and made it into their Instrument Division.
See also *Optometry* 31; Dr. James R. Gregg, O.D. *The Story of Optometry* (NYC: The Ronald Press, 1965) 218, and 219.
Tuition at NICOO was reduced from $50 to $25 in 1899 according to "Terms of Tuition Within Reach of All," *Northern Illinois College of Ophthalmology and Otology* (cat., CHGO: NICOO, 1909).
16. Prof. David Ward Wood, "Dr. George W. McFatrich, of Chicago," OJ, 12:4 (Oct 1903) 516; advertisement OJ Supplement 5:15 (May 15 1899) 131; "The Northern Illinois College of Ophthalmology and Otology," OJ 15:9 (Feb 23 1905) 426-428.
One of Dr. George McFatrich's article series "Subjective and Objective Testing," appeared in OJ 10:1 (Jul 1902) 91-97.
17. Advertisement OJ 5:3 (Mar 15 1899) 67.
18. "Special Announcement," *Northern Illinois College of Ophthalmology and Otology* (cat., CHGO: NICOO, 1905).
19. Advertisement OJ 16:3 (Jul 13 1905); *Optometry* 36.
20. Advertisement OJ 16:3 (Jul 13 1905).
21. Paul Starr, *The Social Transformation of American Medicine.* (NYC: Basic Books, 1982) 57-58 and 102-107.
22. Ibid., 200-215.
23. Dr. James R. Gregg, O.D. *The Story of Optometry* (NYC: The Ronald Press, 1965) 172 and 190; E.E. Arrington, *History of Optometry* (CHGO: White Printing House, 1929) 128.
24. *Opt. Prof.* 132.
25. Ibid.
26. Ibid.,133.
27. Dr. James R. Gregg, O.D., *American Optometric Association: A History* (St.L: AOA, 1972) 10. For an account of the society's establishment and Prentice's courtroom battles see *Opt. Prof.* 134-138.
28. Paul Starr, *The Social Transformation of American Medicine* (NYC: Basic Books, 1982) 223; Dr. James R. Gregg, O.D. *The Story of Optometry* (NYC: The Ronald Press, 1965) 193.
29. H.W. Hofstetter, *Optometry: Professional, Economic, and Legal Aspects* (St.L: The C.V. Mosby Co., 1948) 280.
30. Lens peddlers sold spectacles in remote regions of the continent until well into the 1930s when legislation was finally enacted nationwide. This ended the peddlers' right

to sell spectacles without a qualified health care professional's prescription.
See "Fragments of Optometric History," OW (Mar 17 1949) 394; *Optometry* 19-20.
31. Criticism of optometric education had been voiced for some time such as John C. Eberhardt, "Diploma Mills," OJ 10:1 (Jul 1902) 113.
See also E.E. Arrington, *History of Optometry* (CHGO: White Printing House, 1929) 166-167.
32. Ibid.
33. The AMA's "Medical Education in the United States and Canada," Bulletin #4 by Alexander Flexner (Carnegie Foundation for the Advancement of Teaching, 1910) is commonly referred to today as the Flexner Report.
See H.W. Hofstetter, *Optometry: Professional, Economic, and Legal Aspects* (St.L: The C.V. Mosby Co., 1948) 297; Paul Starr, *The Social Transformation of American Medicine* (NYC: Basic Books, 1982) 118-119.
34. E.E. Arrington, *History of Optometry* (CHGO: White Printing House, 1929) 166-167.
35. Ibid., 168.
36. *Optometry* 30.
37. E.E. Arrington, *History of Optometry* (CHGO: White Printing House, 1929) 113-116.
38. For an account of the association's first meeting see Dr. James R. Gregg, O.D., *American Optometric Association: A History* (St.L: AOA, 1972) 9-10.
See also Dr. James R. Gregg, O.D. *The Story of Optometry* (NYC: The Ronald Press, 1965) 202; Paul Starr, *The Social Transformation of American Medicine* (NYC: Basic Books, 1982) 90-91.
39. Dr. James R. Gregg, O.D., *American Optometric Association: A History* (St.L: AOA, 1972) 32.
40. It is interesting to note that while the debate raged on, optometrists themselves were lodging complaints about the quality of vision care offered by the medical community such as the case history presented in Dr. L.T. Cook, "More Complaints About Oculists," OJ 10:1 (Jul 1902) 118-119.
See also Dr. James R. Gregg, O.D., *American Optometric Association: A History* (St.L: AOA, 1972) 46.
41. Ibid., 51.
42. Ibid., 51-52.
43. Ibid., 65 and 80.
44. Dr. James R. Gregg, O.D. *The Story of Optometry* (NYC: The Ronald Press, 1965) 199-201.
45. Advertisements in OJ 9:4 (Apr 1903) 203; OJ 12:6 (Dec 1903); OJ 8:11 (Nov 1901) 964; OJ 8:9 (Sep 1901) 803.
46. "Instruction by Correspondence," *Northern Illinois College of Ophthalmology and Otology* (cat., CHGO: NICOO, 1905); advertisement OJ 8:5 (May 1901) 591.
47. Ibid.
48. *Focus* 5; advertisement OJ 10:1 (Jul 1902).
49. Accounts of the NICOO's Alumni Association can be found in "The Northern Illinois College of Ophthalmology and Otology," OJ 19:8 (Feb 28 1907) 291; "The McFatrich Clan," OJ (Feb 2 1902) 146; "The Northern Illinois College of Ophthalmology and Otology: Alumni Meeting," OJ 15:10 (Mar 2 1905) 530-532; "Northern Illinois College," OJ 17:10 (Mar 1 1906) 519-520; "Northern Illinois Alumni Association Meeting," OJ 13:4 (Mar 17 1904) 400-401."Northern Illinois College Alumni Meeting," OJ 11:4 (Apr 1903) 414.
50. Ibid.
51. H.W. Hofstetter, *Optometry: Professional, Economic, and Legal Aspects* (St.L: The C.V. Mosby Co., 1948) 297; advertisement OJ&RO 30:25 (Dec 12 1912) 1507.
52. H.W. Hofstetter, *Optometry: Professional, Economic, and Legal Aspects* (St.L: The C.V. Mosby Co., 1948) 309; *Optometry* 32.
53. "Northern Illinois College," *Optometrist and Optician* 5:7 (Sep 1914) 534; "Northern Illinois College," *Optometrist and Optician* 5:11 (Jan 1915) 842.
54. Ibid.
55. Paul Starr, *The Social Transformation of American Medicine* (NYC: Basic Books, 1982) 117; "Honorary Degree for Dr. Colley," *Southtown Economist* (Jun 8 1966); "Credit Where Credit Is Due," IL OP (Sep-Oct 1951) 8.
A female graduate is listed in "Northern Illinois College," OJ&RO 39:19 (May 3 1917) 1240. Female alumni officers, vice-president Mrs. A.M. Henrich and corresponding secretary Ms. Veliquette, are mentioned in "Northern Illinois College," OJ 15:10 (Mar 2 1905) 532; Dr. James R. Gregg, O.D., *American Optometric Association: A History* (St.L: AOA, 1972) 343-344.
56. Letter to Wm. Greenberg from Dr. G.W. McFatrich (Sep 28 1917).
57. "Northern Illinois College Reorganized with New Officers. Chicago School of Refraction Combines with It," OJ&RO 41:1 (Dec 27 1917) 43.
58. Ibid.; *Optometry* 36.
59. Dr. James R. Gregg, O.D. *The Story of Optometry* (NYC: The Ronald Press, 1965) 194.

CHAPTER THREE

1. Transcript of an interview between Dr. James Hasler and Dr. Richard Needles (Oct 16 1990) 1; "Fragments of Optometric History," OW (Mar 17 1949) 404; advertisement OJ Supplement 5:2 (Feb 15 1899) 56; letter from Dr. Richard Needles to Ms Pamela Warbinton (Dec 5 1979) 1.
2. The F.C. Merry Co. eventually became part of the American Optical Co.
See transcript of interview between Dr. James Hasler and Dr. Irvin Borish (Feb 1991) 13-14; transcript of interview between Dr. James Hasler and Dr. Richard Needles (Oct 16 1990) 1; letter from Dr. Richard Needles to Ms Pamela Warbinton (Dec 5 1979) 2; Pamela Warbinton, "A Forgotten Optometry School," *Journal of the Missouri Optometric Association* (2nd quarter 1980) 21.
According to Ms. Warbinton's references in the article, Dr. Needles' teaching credentials at Kansas City School of Optometry are mentioned in Dr. William B. Needles, *I Want to Teach You Optometry* (brochure, Kansas City, MO: Needles Institute of Optometry, 1920).
3. *Focus* 3; advertisement OJ&RO 30:25 (Dec 12 1912) 1507; Dr. James R. Gregg, O.D. *The Story of Optometry* (NYC: The Ronald Press, 1965) 220.
4. *The Blue Book of Optometrists and Opticians* (1922) 22.
5. Drs. William B. Needles and Ernest Occhiena, *Anatomy and Physiology of the Eye* (Kansas City, MO: Needles Institute of Optometry, 1919); Drs. Ernest Occhiena and R.G. Schergens, *Practical Work on the Extrinsic Muscles of the Eye* (Kansas City, MO: Occhiena and Schergens, 1917).

6. Drs. William B. Needles and Ernest Occhiena, *Anatomy and Physiology of the Eye* (Kansas City, MO: Needles Institute of Optometry, 1919) preface.
7. The term "Era of Instrumentation" is used in "Optometry, the Profession," Northern Illinois College of Ophthalmology and Otology (cat., CHGO: NICOO, 1937) 9, and in "Fragments of Optometric History," OW 40:11 (Mar 17 1949) 399.
8. Letter from Dr. Richard Needles to Ms Pamela Warbinton (Dec 5 1979) 3; Carl C. Koch, "William Bray Needles," JAOA 25 (1948) 454.
9. *Optometry* 33; H.W. Hofstetter, *Optometry: Professional, Economic, and Legal Aspects* (St.L: The C.V. Mosby Co., 1948) 310.
10. *Optometry* 34.
11. Dr. Carl F. Shepard ,O.D., "The Shadow of a Tall Man," OW (Jun 17 1948) 830; Dr. Carl F. Shepard, O.D., "Optometric Indoctrination," ICO Newsletter (Nov-Dec 1962) 4; "Dr. Needles to Conduct Northern Illinois College in Addition to Needles Institute," OJ&RO 49: 5 (Feb 2 1922) 55.
12. *Focus* 5.
13. "Dr. Needles to Conduct Northern Illinois College in Addition to Needles Institute," OJ&RO 49:5 (Feb 2 1922) 55.
14. *Blue Book of Optometrists and Opticians* (1922) 22; *Focus* 5; *Northern Illinois College of Optometry* (cat., CHGO: NICO, 1930) 4; "Northern Illinois College and Needles Institute Combined in Larger Quarters in Chicago," OJ&RO 57:14 (Apr 8 1926) 49.
15. Transcript of an interview between Dr. James Hasler and Dr. James Grout (Oct 1990) 3; *Focus* 6.
16. *Focus* 6; *Northern Illinois College of Optometry* (cat., CHGO: NICO, 1930) 4; Dr. James R. Gregg, O.D. *The Story of Optometry* (NYC: The Ronald Press, 1965) 220.
17. Dr. William B. Needles, "Must Optometry Be Stifled," OJ&RO 6:9 (Aug 27 1925) 28.
18. Ibid., 50.
19. Ibid., 29; Dr. James R. Gregg, O.D., *American Optometric Association: A History* (St.L: AOA, 1972) 143-144; Dr. William B. Needles, "Optometry Needs 1,000 Graduates A Year," *A Survey of Optometry in Four Parts* (CHGO: Northern Illinois College of Optometry, 1934) 1.
20. Dr. James R. Gregg, O.D., *American Optometric Association: A History* (St.L: AOA, 1972) 110-111; "Optometry Schools and Colleges Approved by I.A.B.of B.," OJ&RO 64:9 (Aug 30 1929) 26; *Northern Illinois College of Optometry* (cat., CHGO: NICO, 1933); *Focus* 6.
21. *Northern Illinois College of Optometry* (cat., CHGO: NICO, 1937) 10.
22. Ibid., 13.
23. Ibid., 22 and 25-26.
24. Ibid., 22.
25. *Focus* 6.
26. Dr. Richard Needles' letter to Pamela Warbinton (Dec 5 1979) 3.
27. *Northern Illinois College of Optometry* (cat., CHGO: NICO, 1937) 5.
28. Dr. James R. Gregg, O.D. *The Story of Optometry* (NYC: The Ronald Press, 1965) 249-250; "Obituary: Carl F. Shepard, O.D., 1893-1956," AJO 34:1 (Jan 1957) 25.
29. Dr. Shepard took a short hiatus from his post in 1937 when he became dean of the Midwestern College of Optometry (aka: Monroe College of Optometry) for a year. See also "In Memoriam: Dr. Carl F. Shepard—1893-1956," *The Kentucky Optometrist*, 30:10 (Dec 1956) 3; "Shep has Left Us," OW (Nov 22 1956) 2117-2118; "Dr. Carl F. Shepard," JAOA 28:5 (Dec 1956) 301.
30. *Optometry* 37; Dr. E.B. Alexander, "AOA Department Reports Delivered at the 1935 Miami Congress," JAOA 7:3 (Oct 1935) 19.
31. *Optometry* 37.
32. *Northern Illinois College of Optometry* (cat., CHGO: NICO, 1937) 7.
33. Ibid., 8.
34. Ibid.; F.E.G., "Diary of a Modern Interne," *The Focus* (yearbook, CHGO: NICO, 1933) 74.
35. *Glasses* 118-121; Dr. James R. Gregg, O.D. *The Story of Optometry* (NYC: The Ronald Press, 1965) 248.
36. "Fragments of Optometric History," OW (Mar 17 1949) 399.
37. *Northern Illinois College of Optometry* (cat., CHGO: NICO, 1937) 10; F.E.G., "Diary of a Modern Interne," *The Focus* (yearbook, CHGO: NICO, 1933) 75.
38. *Northern Illinois College of Optometry* (cat., CHGO: NICO, 1937) 21.
39. NICO News (Feb 4, 1949); Dr. William B. Needles, "Optometry Needs 1,000 Graduates A Year," *A Survey of Optometry in Four Parts* (CHGO: NICO, 1934) 9.
40. *Northern Illinois College of Optometry* (cat., CHGO: NICO, 1937); F.E.G., "Diary of a Modern Interne," *The Focus* (yearbook, CHGO: NICO, 1933) 75.
41. *Northern Illinois College of Optometry* (cat., CHGO: NICO, 1937) 30.
42. *The Focus* (yearbook, CHGO: NICO, 1933).
43. *The Focus* (yearbook, CHGO: NICO, 1933); *Northern Illinois College of Optometry* (cat., CHGO: NICO, 1937) 3;*Focus* 6.
44. *Northern Illinois College of Optometry* (cat., CHGO: NICO, 1937) 5, 30 and 36-42. According to "Northern Illinois College of Optometry to Hold Commencement Exercises," OW 21:16 (Jun 12 1930) 556, seven women graduated in the June 1930 class.
45. F.E.G., "Diary of a Modern Interne," *The Focus* (yearbook, CHGO: NICO, 1933) 80-81.
46. "From the United States Department of Interior—Guidance Leaflet No. 22," *Optometry* (brochure, CHGO: NICO, 1939).
47. Dr. William B. Needles, "Optometry Needs 1,000 Graduates A Year," *A Survey of Optometry in Four Parts* (CHGO: NICO, 1934); transcript of interview between Dr. James Hasler and Dr. Irvin Borish (Feb 1991) 30.
48. Paul Starr, *The Social Transformation of American Medicine* (NYC: Basic Books, 1982) 272.
49. H.W. Hofstetter, *Optometry: Professional, Economic, and Legal Aspects* (St.L: The C.V. Mosby Co., 1948) 297; Dr. James R. Gregg, O.D., *American Optometric Association: A History* (St.L: AOA, 1972) 152; transcript of interview between Dr. James Hasler and Dr. Irvin Borish (Feb 1991) 42; *Focus*.
50. Dr. James R. Gregg, O.D., *American Optometric Association: A History* (St.L: AOA, 1972) 177; letter from Dr. Richard Needles to Pamela Warbinton (Dec 5 1979) 4.; "Ernest Occhiena—1870-1944," JAOA 16:14 (Nov 1944) 102; letter from Dr. James H. Grout to Dr. James Hasler (Feb 5 1995); Dr. James R. Gregg, O.D., *American Optometric Association: A History* (St.L: AOA, 1972) 206; reprint of Joseph Sullivan, "NICO Statement Regarding Removal of Accreditation," OW 40:24 (Jun 16 1949).
51. H.W. Hofstetter, *Optometry: Professional, Economic, and Legal Aspects* (St.L: The C.V.

Mosby Co., 1948) 296; "Fragments of Optometric History," OW (Mar 17 1949) 406.
52. Otis Graham and Meghan R. Wander, *Franklin D. Roosevelt, His Life and Times: An Encyclopedic View* (NYC: Da Capo Press, 1985).
53. Transcript of an interview between Dr. James Hasler, O.D. and Dr. Frederick Kushner (Oct 1992) 11.
54. Ibid., 11-12.
55. Ibid., 12-13.
56. Ibid., 13-14.
57. *Life's Greatest Possession* (brochure, CHGO: NICO, 1948); "New Home of NICO News," *NICO News* (Sep 1947).
58. *Life's Greatest Possession* (brochure, CHGO: NICO, 1948) 5.
59. *Northern Illinois College of Optometry Bulletin 108* (Oct 1 1947) 7; "Northern Illinois College Discloses Personnel Changes, Building Addition," OW (Dec 25 1947) 1929; *Orientation of New Students* (Oct 14 1948).
60. "Glasses to be Dispensed at Laboratory Cost," *NICO News* 2:2 (Jan 1948) 1.
61. "Northern Illinois College Discloses Personnel Changes, Building Addition," OW (Dec 25 1947) 1929; "Students Applaud 2nd Assembly," NICO News 1:3 (Jan 1947) 1; note from Dr. James H. Grout to Dr. James Hasler (Feb 8 1994).
62. "Northern Illinois College of Optometry," IL OP (Nov-Dec 1950) 16-17; "To the Alumni of Northern Illinois College of Optometry" (May 16 1950).
63. "Pinhole Views," IL OP (Sep-Oct 1950) 6; "Pinhole Views," IL OP (Jul-Aug 1951) 10; "Pinhole Views," IL OP (Jul-Aug 1952) 12.
64. Dr. James R. Gregg, O.D., *American Optometric Association: A History* (St.L: AOA, 1972) 223.

CHAPTER FOUR

1. "Reuben Seid," JAOA 28:1 (Aug 1951) 63; transcript of an interview between Dr. James Hasler, O.D. and Judge Morton Abram (Feb 1991) 2.
2. Transcript of an interview between Dr. James Hasler, O.D. and Judge Morton Abram (Feb 1991) 5, 6, and 48.
3. *Focus* 6.
4. Transcript of an interview between Dr. James Hasler, O.D. and Judge Morton Abram (Feb 1991) 3.
5. *Focus* 6; H.W. Hofstetter, *Optometry: Professional, Economic, and Legal Aspects* (St.L: The C.V. Mosby Co., 1948) 296.
6. *Focus* 6.
7. *Glasses* 11; Dr. James R. Gregg, O.D. *The Story of Optometry* (New York, NY: The Ronald Press, 1965) 252-253.
8. PMMA is more commonly known as plexiglas® or lucite®.
See also *Glasses* 11-13, and 88; Dr. James R. Gregg, O.D. *The Story of Optometry* (NYC: The Ronald Press, 1965) 255-256; Drs. Bernard J. Slatt, M.D., F.R.S.C.(C), and Stein, Harold A., M.D. M.Sc. (Opth), F.R.S.C. (C). *Why Wear Glasses If You Want Contacts? The Story of the New Soft Contact Lenses* (Richmond Hill, Ont., Canada: A Pocket Book Edition, Simon & Schuster of Canada, Ltd., 1972) 11.
9. Dr. James R. Gregg, O.D. *The Story of Optometry* (NYC: The Ronald Press, 1965) 255-256; Drs. Bernard J. Slatt, M.D., F.R.S.C.(C), and Stein, Harold A., M.D. M.Sc. (Opth), F.R.S.C. (C). *Why Wear Glasses If You Want Contacts? The Story of the New Soft Contact Lenses* (Richmond Hill, Ont., Canada: A Pocket Book Edition, Simon & Schuster of Canada, Ltd., 1972) 11.
10. Ibid.
11. *Glasses* 111.
12. Dr. James R. Gregg, O.D., *American Optometric Association: A History* (St.L: AOA, 1972) 184-185; "Fragments of Optometric History," OW (Mar 17 1949) 401.
13. H.W. Hofstetter, *Optometry: Professional, Economic, and Legal Aspects* (St.L: The C.V. Mosby Co., 1948) 133.
14. Norbert Kastner, "Chicago Optometrists Train Vets in Profession," *Illinois Mobilizes for Its Veterans* (May-Jun 1948) 11-12.
15. Transcript of an interview between Dr. James Hasler, O.D. and Judge Morton Abram (Feb 1991) 1-3.
16. Ibid., 6 and 39.
17. Ibid., 4, 6 and 8.
18. Ibid., 8-10.
19. Ibid., 11-15; Drs. Irvin Borish and Eugene Freeman, *Manual of Accrediting of Schools and Colleges of Optometry* (St.L: AOA, 1941) 4-5; "Dr. Wodis New Associate Dean," *Eyes Right* 3:3 (Apr 1949) 1..
20. Ibid., 16.
21. H.W. Hofstetter, *Optometry: Professional, Economic, and Legal Aspects* (St.L: The C.V. Mosby Co., 1948) 297; *Chicago College of Optometry* (cat., CHGO: CCO, 1951) 17 and 32; *Chicago College of Optometry* (cat., CHGO: CCO, 1952) 31 and 29.
22. *Chicago College of Optometry* (cat., CHGO: CCO, 1951) 40.
23. Transcript of an interview between Dr. James Hasler, O.D. and Judge Morton Abram (Feb 1991) 20; "Dean Freeman Pens New Book," *Eyes Right* 6:4 (Apr 1952) 10.
24. Norbert Kastner, "The Road Ahead: A History of Chicago College of Optometry," (yearbook, CHGO: CCO, 1949) 11.
25. Dr. E.R. Tennant, *Introduction to Laboratory Work in Geometrical Optics, 2nd ed.* (CHGO: CCO, 1945); "Dr. Tennant Named Clinic Director," *Eyes Right* 4:4 (Jul 1950) 1; C. Clayton Powell, "Europe's Loss Is CCO's Gain," *Eyes Right* 5:2 (Mar 1951) 4.
26. "Dr. Schoen Joins Faculty," *Eyes Right* 3:3 (Apr 1949) 1; "Pinhole Views: CCO," IL OP (Nov-Dec 1950) 6.
27. Norbert Kastner, "The Road Ahead: A History of Chicago College of Optometry," (yearbook, CHGO: CCO, 1949) 5; "Dr. Murroughs Named Research Director," *Eyes Right* 4:5 (Aug 1950) 1 and 11.
28. Dr. James R. Gregg, O.D., *American Optometric Association: A History* (St.L: AOA, 1972) 169.
29. "Eyes Right Receives First Class Honors Rating," *Eyes Right* 4:3 (May 1950) 1.
30. "The Honor Roll," *Eyes Right* 4:5 (Jan 1950) 5.
31. "Reuben Seid," JAOA (Aug 1951) 63; transcript of an interview between Dr. James Hasler, O.D. and Judge Morton Abram (Feb 1991) 19.

CHAPTER FIVE

1. Richard D. Hazlett and H.W. Hofstetter, "Optometric Education in the United States," JAOA, 38:11 (Nov 1967) 32; "Fragments of Optometric History," OW 40:11 (Mar 17 1949) 401..
2. "Meeting in Minneapolis," *The Alumnus* 5:5-6 (Oct-Dec 1954) 9; Dr. Richard Feinberg, "NICO begins 82nd Year in Education," *The Alumnus* 5:5-6 (Oct-Dec 1954) 3; "Faculty

Adds to Student Fund," *The Alumnus* 5:5-6 (Oct-Dec 1954) 12; Dr. Richard Feinberg, "NICO Moves Ahead—Progress Report," *The Alumnus* 6:4 (Jul-Aug 1954) 17.
3. Dr. Richard Feinberg, "NICO begins 82nd Year in Education," *The Alumnus* 5:5-6 (Oct-Dec 1954) 3; Graduates Since 1940, Illinois College of Optometry Office of the Registrar; "NICO to Have Only One Enrollment Each Year," IL OP (Mar-Apr 1952) 22.
4. In the 1960s, the University of Illinois' Chicago Circle Campus was opened near the medical complex, enlarging the urban renewal project even further; transcript of interview between Dr. James Hasler and Judge Morton Abram (Feb 1991) 21-22.
5. Transcript of interview between Dr. James Hasler and Judge Morton Abram (Feb 1991) 67-68, 23-24; "CCO Associates with Illinois Institute of Technology," *Eyes Right* 7:1 (Oct 1952) 1; "Dr. Abram Heads CCO," *Eyes Right* 7:1 (Oct 1952) 1.
6. Transcript of interview between Dr. James Hasler and Judge Morton Abram (Feb 1991) 24; "Building Program Underway," *Eyes Right* 7:5 (May 1953) 1 and 4; "Chicago College of Optometry," IL OP (May-Jun 1953) 15.
7. "Dr. Abram Wields Shovel in Ground-Breaking," *Eyes Right* 8:4 (Feb 1954) 1 and 11.
8. Transcript of interview between Dr. James Hasler and Judge Morton Abram (Feb 1991) 57.
9. Ibid., 55.
10. Ibid.
11. Ibid., 27-28.
12. *Focus* 7; transcript of interview between Dr. James Hasler and Judge Morton Abram (Feb 1991) 28-29 and 48.
13. *Focus* 7.
14. "Meet Our Faculty," ICO Newsletter (Sep-Oct 1963) 2; "Shuron Salutes Northern Illinois College of Optometry," *Shuron Technician* (Spring 1955) 6; "NICO and CCO Form New Illinois College of Optometry," *The Alumnus* 7 (Summer 1955) 4.
15. "Illinois College of Optometry News," IL OP (Sep-Oct 1955) 19. Dr. Frederick Kushner left the school in 1955 to join Dr. John Brady's in Sheldon, IA. See transcript of interview between Dr. James Hasler and Judge Morton Abram (Feb 1991) 31; "John J. Brady, O.D.," *Who's Who in Optometry* (1963) 2.
16. "First Lady O.D. Receives Army Commission," *ICO Newsletter* 3: (Oct 1961) 2.
17. Richard D. Hazlett and H.W. Hofstetter, "Optometric Education in the United States," JAOA 38:11 (Nov 1967) 932; Graduates Since 1940, Illinois College of Optometry Office of the Registrar.
18. Dr. Frederick Kushner, "Kushner's Korner," *ICO Newsletter* 2:1 (Feb-Mar 1961) 1; "Pinhole Views," IL OP (May-Jun 1955) 8.
19. "President Strawn Welcomes Needles and DeVere as ICO Students," *ICO Newsletter* 4:30 (Jul-Aug 1962) 4.
20. "Public Service Radio Announcements for ICO," *ICO Newsletter* 4:9 (Sep-Oct 1963) 5.
21. Graduates Since 1940, Illinois College of Optometry Office of the Registrar; "ICO Maps Campaign for Endowment Funds," *ICO Newsletter* 3:3 (Nov-Dec 1961) 7; "A Time for Assessment," *ICO Newsletter* (Nov-Dec 1965) 4.; Report of the Dean's Office to the President (Apr 12 1967) 5.
22. ICO Appendix A, 1995 and 1996
23. Dr. James R. Gregg, O.D., *American Optometric Association: A History* (St.L: AOA, 1972) 320-321.
24. Paul Starr, *The Social Transformation of American Medicine* (NYC: Basic Books, 1982) 371-372; Dr. James R. Gregg, O.D., *American Optometric Association: A History* (St.L: AOA, 1972) 311.
25. Paul Starr, *The Social Transformation of American Medicine* (NYC: Basic Books, 1982) 369-370; ICO Appendix A, 1995 and 1996, 9.
26. "ICO Maps Campaign for Endowment Funds," *ICO Newsletter* 3:3 (Nov-Dec 1961) 7.
27. "Speaking Frankly," *ICO Newsletter* 3:2 (Aug-Sep 1961) 3.
28. "ICO Fund Drive Launched," *ICO Newsletter* 4:14 (Jul-Aug 1964); "Building Fund Underway," *ICO Newsletter* 6:1 (Jan-Feb 1965) 1; "ICO Awards Honorary Degrees," *ICO Newsletter* 4:11 (Jan-Feb 1964) 3. W. Clement Stone's *Success Through a Positive Mental Attitude* was published by Prentice-Hall.
29. "Building Fund Underway," *ICO Newsletter* 6:1 (Jan-Feb 1965) 1; "Dedication—Brady Hall," *ICO Newsletter* 4:3 (May-Jun 1965) 3.
30. Dr. Eugene W. Strawn, "The Saga of ICO's Building Permit," *ICO Newsletter* 8:10 (Jul-Aug 1968) 1 and 6-7.
31. Ibid.
32. Dr. Eugene W. Strawn, "Dedication Illinois College of Optometry Eye Clinic and Alumni Memorial Instructional Wing, October 19, 1969," *ICO Newsletter* special (Oct 1969) 1.
33. Ibid.; *Focus* 7.
34. "Dr. Rosenbloom Elected President," OJ&RO 109:8 (Apr 15 1972) 52; "Dr. Rosenbloom Elected President," *ICO Newsletter* 12:4 (Mar-Apr 1972) 1.
35. Report of the Dean's Office to the President (Apr 12 1967) 5; Richard D. Hazlett and H.W. Hofstetter, "Optometric Education in the United States," JAOA 38:11 (Nov 1967) 927; The Dean's Report in Minutes of the Board of Trustees, (Apr 9 1969) 2; ICO Appendix A, 1995 and 1996.
36. *Focus* 1.
37. Ibid.; ICO Appendix A.
38. Dr. James R. Gregg, O.D., *American Optometric Association: A History* (St.L: AOA, 1972) 281 and 284.
39. "ICO Externship Program in Eighth Year," *ICO Newsletter* 7:4 (Jul-Aug 1966) 6.
40. *Focus* 3.
41. Transcript of interview between Dr. James Hasler and Judge Morton Abram (Feb 1991) 31; "A Decade of Progress," *ICO Newsletter* 5:19 (Nov-Dec 1965) 5; "Alumni Gives ICO Three New Clinic Rooms," *ICO Newsletter*, (Nov-Dec 1960); "SC Alumni Chapter Donates Model Examination Room," *ICO Newsletter* (Oct 1961) 2; "Mayor of Chicago Is Guest of Honor at New Clinic Dedication of ICO" *Illinois Optometric Journal* (Jan-Feb 1957) 15; Dean's Report (Apr 9 1969) 3.
42. "Robert R. McCormick Chicago Boys Club Residency Grant," *ICO Newsletter* 4:1 (Jan-Feb 1962) 8.
43. Dr. Leo Manas, "ICO Maze as a Testing Device," *ICO Newsletter* (Mar-Apr 1969) 2 and 4.
44. "New Post for Dr. Jess Goroshow," *ICO Newsletter* 9:4 (Jul-Aug 1969) 2; *Focus* 8.
45. *Focus* 8; "Dr. Rosenbloom Elected ICO President," OJ&RO 109:8 (Apr 15 1972) 52; "Dr. Weinstein Elected Acting President Announces Appointment," *ICO Newsletter* 12:3 (Jan-Feb 1972) 1.

46. *A Newer World to See* (ICO Centennial Program, 1972); Dr. James R. Gregg, O.D., *American Optometric Association: A History* (St.L: AOA, 1972) 307.
47. "The College of Tomorrow," *A Newer World to See* (ICO Centennial Program, 1972).
48. "Project Director Named for HEW Grant," *ICO Newsletter* (Jan-Feb 1973) 4; "New ICO Staff Promotions and Faculty Additions," *ICO Newsletter* 13:5 (Sep-Oct 1973) 4.
49. The scholarship was funded by the Drexel National Bank, a South Side bank whose President, Norman Alperin was an ICO trustee and board president.
See "Mrs. Carletta Boyd Awarded 'Promise to Go Back' Scholarship," *ICO Alumni Newsletter* 13:5 (Sep-Oct 1973) 8.
50. Dr. James R. Gregg, O.D., *American Optometric Association: A History* (St.L: AOA, 1972) 310.
51. "Underprivileged Saved by Vision Project," *ICO Newsletter* (Jan-Feb 1972) 10; "ICO Opens Off-Campus Clinic," *ICO Alumnus* (Jan-Feb 1974) 5.
52. "ICO Opens Off-Campus Clinic," ICO Alumnus (Jan-Feb 1974) 5.
53. The National Optometric Association was organized in the days of Jim Crow segregation by African-American optometrists who were denied AOA entry. The AOA was no longer segregated in 1972, but the NOA remained active.
See also "ICO Welcomes Class of 1977," *ICO Alumnus* 13:5 (Sep-Oct 1973) 1; "ICO Named College of the Year," *JAOA* (Sep-Oct 1973) 21.
54. "ICO Students included in Indiana VOSH Mission," *ICO Alumni Newsletter* (Jan-Feb 1977) 3.
55. Report from Dr. Yasko in the *ICO Alumni Newsletter* (Jan-Feb 1974.) 9.
56. ICO Appendix A, 1995 and 1996.
The 1986 amendment of the federal Social Security Act to provide for parity and equity in reimbursements, under Part B of the Medicare Program, for optometrists with physicians (e.g. ophthalmologists) for services provided by optometrists.
57. Paul Starr, *The Social Transformation of American Medicine* (NYC: Basic Books, 1982) 396 and 415.
58. Paul Starr, *The Social Transformation of American Medicine* (NYC: Basic Books, 1982) 420-421.
59. "ICO Conducts Contact Lens Research," *ICO Alumnus* (Jan-Feb 19??) 5.
60. "Pediatric Optometry Department Expands," *ICO Alumni Newsletter* (Jan-Feb 1978); Report to the President on Institutional Research 1974-1975.
61. "Pediatric Optometry Department Expands," *ICO Alumni Newsletter* (Jan-Feb 1978).
62. Dr. Michael D. Shansky, Ph.D., "Report to the President on Institutional Research, 1974-75," in President's Report to the Board of Trustees, Oct 1974; "150 Enter ICO Class of 1979," *ICO Alumnus* (Sep-Oct 1975) 1.
63. "Wesley-Jessen Leader in Contact Lens Development," *Image* (Spring 1995) 8-9.
64. "ICO Acquires VER Computer," *ICO Alumni Newsletter* (Jan-Feb 1976).
65. ICO Board of Trustees Announces Administration Reorganization and Presidential Search, 1981; "Dr. Rosenbloom to Retire as ICO President But Will Become Distinguished Prof," *AOA News* (Nov 15 1981); "Nizza Named Clinic Director," *ICO Alumnus* (May-Jun 1978); "Conway and Petty Join ICO Staff," *ICO Alumnus* (Oct-Dec 1979) 1; "Dr. Grosvenor Named New Academic Head," *ICO Alumnus* (May-Jun 1977) 1.

CHAPTER SIX

NOTE: Most of the material found in this chapter comes from a document entitled ICO Appendix A. Other references are noted below.
1. Transcript of an interview between Dr. Boyd B. Banwell and the authors (Nov 1995) 1.
2. *Illinois College of Optometry* (cat.: CHGO: ICO, 1994) 53.
3. Ibid.
4. This examination is presently only required by 36 states in lieu of a state practical examination. The remaining states require Part Two in addition to a state-administered proficiency examination.
5. The Association of Schools and Colleges of Optometry's 1995 Annual Survey of Optometric Educational Institutions reported that the nation's professional schools had 53.6 percent female enrollment, and 46.4 percent male enrollment.
See also "Women in Optometry," *Image* 18:2 (Summer 1995) 16-17.
6. "Profile: Millicent Knight," *Image* 18:2 (Summer 1995) 8-9 and 19.
7. Ibid.
8. "ICO Featured in JAOA," *Image* (Winter 1994) 12; Stuart Richer, M.S., O.D., "Guest Editorial: Atrophic ARMD — a Nutrition Responsive Chronic Disease," *JAOA* 76:1 (Jan 1996) 6-10.
9. Transcript of an interview between Dr. Boyd B. Banwell and the authors (Nov 1995) 23.
10. "Gerald R. Ford to Speak at Installment Ceremony," *Image* 4:2 (Spring 1983) 1.
11. Ibid.
12. "New Appointments Announced," *ICO Alumni* (Nov-Dec 1974) 4.
13. Transcript of an interview between Dr. Boyd B. Banwell and the authors (Nov 1995) 20.
14. By 1988, DPA legislation had been enacted nationwide. Recent legislation allows the utilization of therapeutic pharmaceutical agents (TPAs). State educational requirements nationwide dictate that optometrists might first be certified in the use of DPAs and then successfully complete 120 classroom hours in the clinical use of TPAs at an accredited optometric college. New graduates wishing to use DPAs and TPAs must obtain certification at the time of their initial licensure.
See also "Illinois Number 45 with TPA Rights," *Image* 18:2 (Summer 1995) 3.
15. Transcript of an interview between Dr. Boyd B. Banwell and the authors (Nov 1995) 27-28.
16. Ibid.
17. Ibid.
18. "Name Dr. Greenberg VP/Dean," *Image* 6:5 (Dec 1984) 1.
19. Ibid.
20. "New ICO Trustees Named," *ICO Alumnus* 14:11 (Jan-Feb 1974) 1.
21. "Optometry's Flagship," *JAOA* 65:5 (May 1994) 30.
22. "ICO Plays Key Role in Fragile X Clinic," *Image* 17:3 (Autumn 1994) 6-9.
23. "ICO Develops Innovative Eye Care Program for Easter Seal Society," *ICO Alumni Magazine* (DATE?) 18-19.
24. "Spotlight on Sports Vision," *Image* 13:6 (Dec 1990) 9-10.
25. Ibid.; "Sports Vision and ICO" *Image* 9:4 (Aug 1988) 1.

26. Transcript of interview between Dr. Br. Boyd B. Banwell and the authors (Nov 1995) 4-6 and 21.
27. Ibid. 21.
28. Ibid.

INDEX

Abram, Morton, 66-67, 70-73, 82-84
Adams Center, 127
Advanced Ophthalmic Care, 118, 127
affirmative action, 94, 96
African-American, 73, 95, 116
Albizu Campos Center, 95
Albrittain, J.W., 92
Alhazen, 3
Allen Cars, 103
Alpha Chapter of Phi Kappa Rho, 54
Alumni Association, 34-35, 81-, 84-85, 88, 92
Alumni Memorial Instructional Wing, 89
American Academy of Optometry, 94-107, 109-110
American Association of Optometry, 94, 107, 109-110
American Association of Opticians, 31-32
American Institute of Architects, 124
American Medical Association (AMA), 25, 38, 30-32, 44, 51, 56, 60
American Ophthalmological Society, 12
American Optical Company, 14
American Optometric Association (AOA), 32, 36, 43, 46, 56, 59, 70-72, 76, 83, 91-92, 94-95, 106, 109, 112, 116
American Optometric Foundation, 90
Amoco Foundation, 119
Amundsen, Roald, 69
Aristotle, 4
Armati, Salvino d', 4
ARMD atrophic, 110-111
Army, U.S., 70, 77, 85
Art of Seeing, The, 51
Ashby, Hugh, 89
Asian-American, 95
Atkinson, Dr. Thomas G., 50
Audemaire Trial Case, 24
Australia, 34
Austria, 57-58, 67, 73
B.S.V.S., 106
Babbage, Charles, 13
Bachelor of Ophthalmology, 33; of Optics 35; of Science, 44, 106, 112
Bacon, Roger, 4
Banks, Ernie, 97
Bartisch, Georg, 9-10
Bates Method, 51
Bates, Dr. William H., 51
Bayley, Scales, 103
Beckerman, Dr. Stephen, 120
Benito Juarez Clinic, 95
Bennett College of Medicine, 19-20, 23
Bennett, Dr. H.F., 24
Berkeley, University of California at, 43-44
Berkenheimer, Earl R., 77
Bernhard Hotel, 54-55
Bill H.D. 7966, 91
Boger, Frederick, 31
Book of Optics, The, 3
Borish, Dr. Irvin, 50-51, 56
Boston University, 106
Boyd, Carletta, 95
Brady Hall, 88, 127
Brady, Dr. John J., 82, 85, 88

Brandt, Dr. John E., 116
Brazil, 110
British Optical Association, 28
Brodnax, Dr. Junius, 73
Brown, Olive, 51
Butler University, 77
Butler, Dr. James, 116
California State Board of Optometry, 55
Canada, 30, 34; Canadian, 13, 30
Cardinal Nino de Guevara, 9
Caribbean, 97, 110
Carnegie Foundation, 30
Causanus, Nicholas, 4-5
centennial, 94-95
Chapman, Dr. W. Judd, 116
Chicago College of Optometry (CCO), 65, 67, 70-77, 82-85, 100, 105
Chicago: Art Institute, 77; Bulls, 121; Housing Authority, 124; Lighthouse for the Blind, 97; Museum of Science and Industry, 97; Post-Graduate Optical College, 24; School of Refraction, 37; Strabismus Project, 74, 76; White Sox, 120
children, 49, 93, 95, 97-98, 117, 120
China, 1, 69; Chinese, 3-4
Civil Service Commission, 86
Code of Ethics, 46, 70
College of Du Page, 120
Colley, Dr. Ellen, 36
Columbia University, 34, 37., 43, 109
Combined American Insurance Co., 88
continuing education, 32, 92, 108-109, 116, 127
Conway, Shane J., 100
Cook County: Bureau of Public Welfare, 52; Hospital. 20, 23, 82
Corbett, Margaret, 51
Costa Rica, 109
Council of Education (COE), 106-107, 111, 115
COVD, 110
Cross, Dr. Andrew J., 28, 31-31, 34
Cuba, 25
Cuff, John, 10
Culpepper, Nicholas, 10
Cure of Imperfect Sight, The, 51
Daley, Richard J., 92-93
Dames Club, 75-76
De Berillo, 5
De Paul University, 70, 120
Department: of Ethics, 50; of Medical Education, 108; of Psychology, 50
Department, Chicago: of Streets, 89
Department, U.S.: of Defense, 86; of Health, 86; of Health, Education, and Welfare (HEW), 86-87; of National Affairs, 86; of Transportation, 86
DeVere, David, 86; Dr. Paul N., 86
Distinguished Professor of Optometry, 101

District of Columbia, 37
Doctor of Ophthalmology, 33, 35; of Optics, 33, 35; of Optometry, 45, 91
Downs Syndrome, 117
DPAs (diagnostic pharmaceutical agents), 91, 109, 113
Duryea, David, 96
Dynamic Ocular Tests, 32
Easter Seal Society of Metropolitan Chicago, 119, 126
Ebbeson, Dr. Joseph B., 116
Egan, Dr. Howard, 59
Egyptians, 3
Einhorn, Neil, 96
El Greco, 9
Elite Test Case, 24
Ellis, Dr. Carl, 95
England, 5, 155; English, 46, 57-58
enrollment, 34, 36, 42, 48, 55-57, 67, 82, 85-86, 88, 95, 108-109
Era of Instrumentation, 41, 43
Erie House Clinic, 95
Eton, 51
Euclid, 4
Europe, 5, 9, 17, 57-58; European, 4, 7-9, 14, 43, 58, 68,
Evans House, 76
Ewalt, H. Ward, 71
Eyebright, 10
Eyemen, The, 76
Eyes-Right, 76
Family Relief Association, 52
Farr, Newton, 83
Federhar, Richard H., 77
Feinberg, Dr. Richard, 60, 83-85
Feinbloom, Dr. William, 68
Ferris State University, 112
Fick, Dr. A. Eugen, 67
First World War, 36, 43
Flexner, Alexander, 30
Florida, 70, 116; Florida Optometric Association, 116
Focus, The, 47, 54
Fragile X Syndrome, 117-118
France, 5, 10-11; French, 11
Franklin, Benjamin, 10-11
Freeman, Dr. Eugene, 56, 73, 82
Friedlander, Dr. Edward, 59
Funk, Williston C., 77
G.I. Bill, 57, 70, 6-77
Galen, 4
Good will Agency, 52
Goroshow, Dr. Jess E., 89, 94
Great Britain, 12, 28, 57
Great Lakes U.S. Naval Hospital, 92
Greece, 4; Greeks, 3
Greenberg, Dr. David A., 110, 115-116
Greenberg, Wm., 36
Grout, Dr. James, 59
Guatemala, 109
Gutenberg, 2-3
Hahnemann Medical College, 19
Haiti, 96, 99
Hall, Otis F., 22-23
Hampden, Walter, 68
Hamu, Barbara, 116
Hauser, Dr. Samuel, 66

147

Health Professions Educational Assistance Act, 86, 88
Heather, Dr. W. Jerome, 48, 50, 52-53
Henry, Dr. Joseph L., 112-113, 116
Hicks, George, 71
Hill, Dr. C.K., 88, 113, 116
Himley, Karl, 11
Hispanic-American, 95
HMOs, 26, 98, 107
Hoffmann, Dr. Bernard, 50-51
Hollywood, 68-69
Howard University School of Dentistry, 116
Hull House, 52
Huxley, Aldous, 51
Hyde Park YMCA, 54
Hydrolens, 98
Illinois College of Optometry (ICO), 2, 26, 41, 45, 56, 58, 65, 81, 84-85, 88, 91-93, 97, 102, 105, 108, 115-116
Illinois Division of Rehabilitation, 70
Illinois Emergency Relief, 52
Illinois Eye Institute (IEI), 85, 89, 92, 95, 97-98, 100, 109-110, 116-121, 125-127
Illinois Institute of Technology (IIT), 73, 82-83, 88, 120
Illinois Masonic Medical Center, 126
Illinois Optometric Association, 97
Illinois Optometric Practice Act, 113
Illinois Optometric Society, 36-37
Illinois Senate Bill, 185, 112
Illinois State Board of Examiners, 109
Illinois Visually Handicapped Institute, 96
Indian Health Service, 86
Indiana, State Prison, 96
Indiana University, 96
Institute of Ophthalmic Opticians, 28
International Association of Board of Examiners, 44
International Board of Boards (IBB), 44-47, 56, 67
Inuit, 69
Jessen, Dr. George, 100
Job Corps, 95
Johnson, C. Porter, 24
Johnson, William A., 92
Johnston Optical Institute, 19
Jordan, Michael, 121
Juvenile Court, 52
Kaiser Plan, 98
Kalt, Edouard, 67
Kansas City School of Optometry, 42
Kennedy, Dr. John, 85
Kennedy, Senator Edward M., 87
Keystone View Co., 49
King Optical Co., 24
Kirchner, James, 96
Knight Architects Engineers Planners, Inc., 127
Knight, Dr. Millicent, 109-110
Kohn, Harold, 71
Korean War, 85

Kushner, Dr. Frederick R., 57-58, 85-86, 92, 113, 116; "Kushner's Korner," 85
LaPaz Child Development Center, 96
Latin American, 110
Lichenlack, Lillian, 89
Lions Club, 95
Little City Eye Clinic, 96
Little League, 120
Louisiana Polytechnic Institute, 77
Loyola University, 50, 59, 120
Macular Degeneration Study Group, 110
Manas, Dr. Leo, 76, 92-93, 102
Manual of Accrediting Schools and Colleges, 56
Marshall, Dr. Walter, 97
Martin Bell Syndrome, 117
Maryville Academy, 95, 120
Master of Ophthalmology, 33; of Science, 19
Maybee, Elva, 37
Mayo Clinic, 1111
McAllister, James, 10
McCormick Boys Club, Robert R., 93, 95
McCormick Optical College, 19, 41
McCormick, Dr. Charles, 41
McFatrich, 19-20, 22-25, 33-34, 36-37, 44-45; Eye,33; Dr. George Wilbur, 20, 23-24, 36-37, 44-45; Dr. James Burton, 19-20, 22, 34
McGuire, Dr. C. Stanley, 58
Medicaid, 87, 112
Medicare, 87
men, 22, 31, 46, 48, 55, 67, 69-70, 84-85, 117
Merry Company, F.C., 42
Metcalfe, Ralph, 96
Michael Reese Hospital Medical Center, 65, 82
Michigan Optometry Association, 112
Midwestern College of Optometry, 112
Minnesota law, 28-30, 32
Minority Recruitment, 95-96
Monroe College of Optometry (MCO), 66-67, 70-71, 84-85 100
Montreal Expos, 120
Moore, Dr. Glenn H., 84
Mt. Sinai Hospital Medical Center, 116
Mullen, John, 68
Murine Eye Remedy Co., 22-23, 44
Murroughs, Dr. Thaddeus, 71, 76, 93
National Board of Examiners (NBEO), 107-108, 110
National Eye Institute, 100
National Optometric Association (NOA), 96
National Organization of State Boards of Examiners, 32
Native-American, 68, 95
Navy, U.S., 70, 77
Needles, 41-46, 48-49, 56-57, 59-60, 65-66, 86, 90; Dr. Richard, 48, 59-60; Dr. William Bray, 41-46, 49, 56, 59, 65-66, 90; Institute of

Optometry, 42, 45, 49; Philip, 86
Neighborhood Youth Corps, 95
Nelson, Dr. Peter, 95
New England College of Optometry, 115
New York Medical Society, 27
New Zealand, 34
Nizza, Dr. Anthony, 100
North Central Association of Schools and Colleges, 106; Colleges and Secondary Schools, 90
Northern Illinois College of Ophthalmology and Otology (NICOO), 17, 20, 22-23, 26, 29-30, 33-34, 36-37, 41, 44-51, 53-60, 65-67
Northern Illinois College of Optometry (NICO), 45-51, 53-60, 66-67, 73, 76-77, 81-86, 88, 90, 93, 105, 112
Northern Illinois Eye Clinic, 49-51, 53, 59, 85; Northern Illinois Eye Institute, 92
Northwestern University, 95
Noyes, Dr. Henry D., 27
Nugent, Luci Johnson, 94
Nuremberg High Council, 7
Oak Park Easter Seal Society, 95
Obrig, Theodore, 68
Occhiena, Dr. Ernest, 42-43, 45, 49, 53, 57
oculists, 11-12, 28, 45
Office of Equal Opportunity (OEO), 87
Ogawa, Toshimi, 77
Ohio State University, 32; College of Optometry, 74
Olin, Dr. Henry, 19-20
Olivier, Sir Laurence, 68
ophthalmologists, 11-12, 29, 45-46, 90, 107, 113, 115
ophthalmology, 9, 11, 17, 19-20, 22, 24, 33, 35-36, 44, 95
Ophthalmos, Inc. 98
Optical Journal and Review of Optometry, 31, 37, 44
Optical Journal, 22, 24, 31, 37, 44-45
Optical Society of the State of new York (OSSNY), 31
Optical Truths, 42
opticians, 10-13, 22-23, 27-29, 31-32
optics, 2-3, 5, 9, 14, 22, 24, 29, 33, 35-36, 47, 73
Optometric College Aptitude Tests (OCAT), 86
Optometric Extension Program, 49
Optometric Weekly, 49
optometrists, 1-2, 29, 31, 42-47, 55-56, 58-59, 67, 69-70, 76-77, 81, 85-87, 89, 91, 95-96, 98, 105-109, 112-113, 115, 119-120, 125-126, 128
Opus Major, 4
orthoptics, 49, 51-52
Paris Exposition, 14
Parker, Dorothy, 69
pediatric, 50, 81, 93-94, 99, 102, 109, 117-119, 126-127; Clinic, 50, 99, 102
Peterson, John, 98
Philip, Nancy, 116

INDEX

Phoenicians, 3
physicians, 3, 9-12, 26-27, 30, 34, 56, 87
physics, 29, 48, 50
physiology, 19, 24, 29, 42-43, 47, 50, 99
ping-pong, 24
Plastic Constant lens Co., 100
Plato, 73
PMMA, 68
Polaroid, 69
Politzer, Michael, 98
Polo, Marco, 1, 4
Powell, Dr. C. Clayton, 96
Prentice, Charles F., 27, 34
Prentice, Dr. Chalmers, 24, 27
President, U.S.: Ford, Gerald R., 111, 113; Jefferson, Thomas, 10; Johnson, Lyndon B., 87, 94; Kennedy, John F., 86-87; McKinley, William, 25; Roosevelt, Franklin D., 56; Roosevelt, Theodore, 25
Project Head Start, 94-95
Promise to Go Back, 95, 113
psychology, 24, 26, 29, 47, 50, 74, 91
Ptolemy, 4
public health service, 96
Ransdell, Dr. Ward R., 116
Raphael, 4
Reiser, Dr. Stanley, 107
Retaliato, John T., 82
Rhode Island, 91
Richer, Dr. Stuart, 110
Rodriguez, Dr. Albert, II, 116
Rogers, Dr. George A., 24, 37
Roggenkamp, Dr. John, 93, 98
Roman, 3
Roosevelt, College, 77; University, 77
Rosenbloom, Dr. Alfred A., 89-2, 94, 101
Ross Professor of Humanities, 107
Ruby, Dr. George B., 50
Rush Medical College, 107
Rush Presbyterian-St. Luke Hospital, 82, 118, 120
Sacred Heart Church, 52
Salvation Army, 52
Schoen, Dr. Z. John Bruce, 74
School of Public Health, 108
Second World War, 52, 56, 58-59, 67, 68, 70, 81, 108, 112
Seid, Dr. Reuben, 65-67, 70-71, 73, 77, 82
Sharp, John, 98
Sheard, Dr. Charles 32
Shepard, Dr. Carl F., 49, 59-60, 66
Sherman, Lawrence Y., 25
Shonka, Dr. Francis, 59
Shulman, Dr. Paul F., 92
Siberian, 69
Siemsen, Dr. Dennis W., 106-107
SILO response, 99
Sirutus, H., 9
Skeffington, Dr. A.M., 49-50
Slaughter, Oliver, 95
Slaymaker, Second Lt. Freda J., 85
Snellen, Herman, 63

Social Security Administration, 87
Solex Laboratories, 69
South America, 34, 97
South Carolina Alumni Chapter, 92
Spain, 9; Spanish, 9, 69
Spanish-American War, 25
Spencer Optical Institute, 24
Spina, Brother Alessandro della, 4
Spitz, Warren, 83
Sports Vision, 120-121, 125
St. Jerome, 7
St. John Roosa, Dr. D.B., 27
State: of Illinois, 20, 33; of New York, 28, 31
Stone, W. Clement, 58, 88, 93
strabismus, 51-52, 74, 76, 93, 99, 117
Strawn, Dr. Eugene, 66-67, 84, 89-90, 94, 125
sunglasses, 67, 69
Supreme Court, 31
surgery, 2-3, 19, 51, 115, 118; surgeons, 6
Supreme Court, 31
surgery, 2-3, 19, 51, 115, 118; surgeons, 6
Takahashi, Dr. Ernest S., 73
Tennant, Dr. E.R., 67, 71, 73, 85
Thompson, James, 125
Titmus Color Test, 98
TPA (therapeutic pharmaceutical agents), 112-113
Tucker, Dr. Henry S., 24
Tuohy, Kevin, 69
Turner, Dr. C.D., 59
U.S.: Congress 57, 87; Indian, 110; FDA, 100; Olympic, 120; Patent 19
United Charities, 52
United Way, 119
University: of Arizona, 77; of Buffalo, 74; of California, 43-44; of Chicago Laboratory School, 120; of Chicago, 33, 59, 90, 120; of Hawaii, 77; of Illinois, 65, 82, 108, 120; of Miami, 77; of Rochester, 60; of Texas Health Sciences Center, 107; of Vienna, 57-58; of Virginia, 74
Upper Iowa University, 19
Upward Bound, 95
Use of Spectacles, 9-10
Valdes, Benito Daza de, 9
Vandercook College of Music, 125
Vanderfelz, Don, 96
Veterans Administration, 86, 124
veterans, 52, 57, 70, 76, 86, 91, 95, 124
Vienna, 57-58; Viennese, 73
Vietnam War, 95
Vision Project, 95
Visual Analysis Handbook, 93
Visual Science, 14, 100, 106
von Helmholz, Herman Ludwig Ferdinand, 13-14
VOSH, 96-97, 99, 109-110
W.K. Kellogg Foundation National Fellowship Program, 110
Washington Square Health Foundation, 119

Wayne State University, 112
Weinstein, Dr. O.W., 94
Wesley, Dr. Newton, 100
Wesley-Jessen, 100
Wheeler, Rev. J. Kittredge, 24
Wodis, Dr. Hyman S., 66-67, 71, 85, 89
Wolfe, Benjamin S., 116
Woll, Frederic A., 34
women, 34, 36, 48, 52, 54, 69, 76, 85, 94-95, 117
Woolf, Dr. Howard J., 116
Worshipful Company of Spectaclemakers, 7, 10, 28
Yasko, Dr. Walter, 85, 89, 92, 96-97
Zoethout, Dr. W.D., 45, 50

149

This book was designed and produced by Anistatia R Miller and Jared M. Brown on a Mactinosh 145B Powerbook using Quarkexpress 3.3 software. The text of this book was set in Century Old Style with bold and italics. The captions were set in Futura. The chapter titles were set in Linnotype Didot.

All photographs were supplied courtesy of the Illinois College of Optometry and Al Pouch with the exception of the Inuit snow goggles which are courtesy of the authors and the University of British Columbia Museum of Anthropology in Vancouver, British Columbia, Canada.

Color separations, printing, and bindery were supplied by Dai Nippon Printing Co., Inc., Tokyo Japan. All pages were printed on U-lite matte #86.

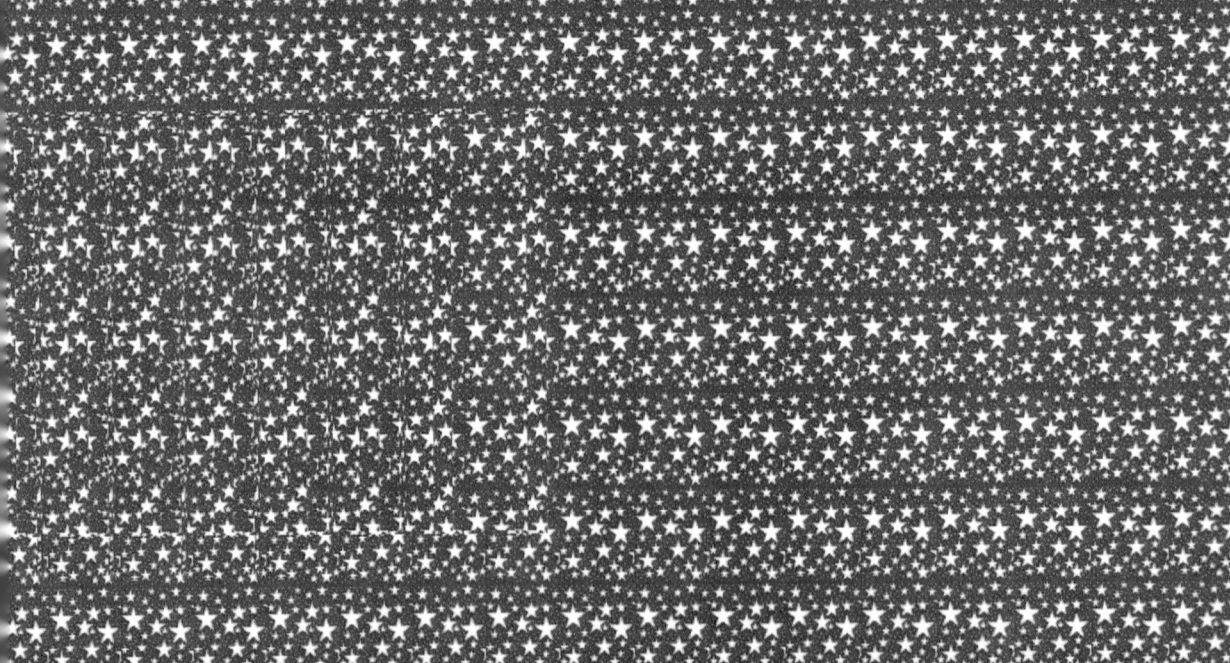